The ANY diet diary

M. Evans and Company, Inc.
~New York~

M. Evans and Company, Inc.
216 East 49th Street
New York, NY 10017

ISBN 0-87131-865-2 9 (paper)

Design by Karlin Gray

Manufactured in the United States of America

9 8 7 6 5 4 3 2 1

HOW TO USE THE ANY DIET DIARY

GETTING STARTED

The first section of this diary provides the "YOU ARE HERE" point on your roadmap to success. A realistic view of where you are, what you want to accomplish, and your plan of how to implement change and achieve your goal is essential.

ASSESSMENT (pages 4-5)

Record your current eating habits. Be sure to include all aspects of how, when, and what you eat. Don't forget to also include your "good" eating habits. Now carefully and honestly review what you've just written and decide what you want to change. Are you only changing the foods you eat or should your changes include elements of when and how you eat? Record the eating behaviors you want to change.

Next, document your plan. This should include the specifics of the diet plan you have chosen, as well as related behavior changes that need to be made, such as "Be sure to eat breakfast" or "No more eating in the car." Sometimes it is actually behavior that needs correction before better food choices can be made.

Now, turn your attention to your physical activity level, or the lack thereof. Enter your current activity level including physical aspects of your daily life. Do not make the mistake of overestimating the physical benefit of daily life activities. Most dieter's find increased exercise plays an invaluable role in any weight loss or health plan and volumes of research support this experience. What is your desired level of physical activity? What is the specific exercise plan you intend to follow?

Next, you will find a space to record your current or beginning weight, followed by a space to record your desired weight. Weight is one of the most often debated subjects in dieting and health. When to weigh, what you should weigh, how fast, how slow, the list goes on and on. Many diet plans come with instructions on how and when to weigh, and as this diary is designed to be used with any plan, the instruction here, is to be consistent. Use the same scale each time you record your weight, wear the same type of clothing (or none at all), and weigh each time at the same time of day. Weigh if you find it helpful to weigh, as a motivator to keep you on track.

Weight is frequently given too much recognition for measuring progress while dieting. Other important measurements include inches lost and/or how your clothing fits. You will find a space to write in measurements of your chest, waist, hips, and thigh. If it is awkward to measure these areas yourself, get some assistance. Be sure to measure each area consistently in future assessment pages providing an accurate record of your progress. Remember to measure only one thigh and continue to measure the same one! Also, note the measurements you desire. Be realistic, be bold, go for it!

Next, is clothing size. Again, document your beginning and desired sizes. Many people who don't like to weigh, depend on this particular yardstick to measure success.

Now, summarize what you want to change, which may include your weight, a particular area of your body, a health concern, your energy or activity endurance level, or other issues important to you concerning your health and appearance. Emotional factors can also be helpful to record. How do you feel about your appearance, self-esteem, health, activity and fitness level, and general outlook on life? What commitments are you willing to make to put a plan into action? There are no wrong answers here! Be honest and be bold! Many times we modify what we truly want because we are afraid that we can't have it, but intense desire is an important motivator, so be honest. What do you really want and what changes are you willing to make?

GOALS

Get specific! The better you can see a target, the better your chance of hitting it! This section records your desire in actual terms. Do you want to weigh a specific weight or do you want to lose weight to a range you can accept? Do you want specific numbers as goals for your measurements? What about your health and fitness goals? Do you have a specific idea of how you want to look and feel? Give this some serious thought and write it down. Make a commitment.

PLAN

Write out the full plan you have chosen to achieve your goals. You can record any and all elements that make up your plan. The diet and exercise plan you noted above, behavior changes and how you will make them, and any nutritional supplements you plan to use. Writing out the details of your plan is important. It records your understanding of the plan and your commitment to the plan.

DAILY DIARY PAGE

These pages are designed to give you maximum flexibility. Write in the day of the week, the date and the day number of your diet. If for any reason you want to start over or change your diet plan while progressing, you have the flexibility to note how many days you have followed that particular plan or portion of the plan.

You will notice that the daily page separates BREAKFAST, LUNCH, DINNER, and SNACKS. Note the time you eat each meal and enter the individual foods or dishes you eat in the space provided. Remember to record everything you consume, including sauces, condiments, beverages, etc. There is also a space for the amount—be sure to document how much you've eaten, as this is essential in figuring food values. Each meal has a space to record water intake. Water is vitally important on any diet and make sure that you record how many glasses you drink each day.

The charts provided allow you to calculate the appropriate food value counts related to any diet that you may be following. Diets vary greatly in philosophy and different diets require you to count different items. This space allows you to record what is pertinent to the diet plan you are following so use this space appropriately. You can look up the related counts in the extensive directory at the back of this book and refer to appropriate food labels as well. Many people record these counts as they write down the foods they've eaten, while others do it at the end of the day. Any system will work, just make sure you record what is relevant to your diet. There is also a space for daily totals.

Exercise and daily activities are equally important and you will want to note them daily. Include the activity, the time of the activity and the quantity, or duration, of the exercise or activity.

Many people include vitamins and supplements in their diet plans and you can note these as well on your daily diary sheets, again noting the time and quantity.

A smiley face rating system is located on each daily diary page to sum up how you felt about today's progress as well as to identify when you need to do better. Use it to motivate and reward yourself and to notice if you would like to renew your commitment and start fresh tomorrow.

The notes section is for you to write whatever you want: how did you feel? what affected you? what did you want to eat that you stayed away from? what did you achieve that is significant to you? how did you reward yourself? what additional commitments need to be made and how will you go forward tomorrow?

WEEKLY ASSESSMENT PAGES
These pages provide the same assessment information you completed at the beginning of the diet. Use these to chart your weekly progress. Be sure you are consistent so your comparisons are accurate, allowing appropriate adjustments to be made in your plan.

COMPLETE NUTRITIONAL VALUES
This invaluable resource is right at your fingertips. Over 2,000 foods are documented with calorie, fat, protein, carbohydrate, cholesterol, sodium, and fiber counts, providing you with one resource to carry at all times, allowing the most comprehensive, convenient recording of your eating patterns.

WHERE DO I BEGIN?

Current eating habits (skip meals, eat late at night, typical foods):

_____

_____

Eating behaviors I want to change:

_____

_____

Diet or eating plan I have chosen:

_____

_____

Current physical activity:

_____

_____

Desired physical activity:

_____

_____

Physical activity plan:

_____

_____

	BEGINNING	DESIRED	ACHIEVED
MEASUREMENTS Chest	46	38-40	
Waist	44	34	
Hips	53	40-42	
Thigh	31	21	

	BEGINNING	DESIRED	ACHIEVED
CLOTHING SIZE Shirt	1X-2X	14	
Pant	22	14	
Dress	22	14	
Belt			

Beginning Weight: _____

Desired Weight: _____

Notes: _____

_____

_____

_____

_____

_____

_____

Desired Daily Totals

CALORIES	FAT	CARBS	PROTEIN	CHOLESTEROL	SODIUM	FIBER

PHOTOS

Date: _____

Day #: _____

Weight: _____

Size: _____

COMMITMENT PHOTO:

Ready to begin!

Date: _____

Day #: _____

Weight: _____

Size: _____

PROGRESS PHOTO:

Motivated and seeing results!

PHOTOS

Date: _____
Day #: _____
Weight: _____
Size: _____

**PROGRESS
PHOTO:**

*Determined
to succeed!*

Date: _____
Day #: _____
Weight: _____
Size: _____

**CELEBRATION
PHOTO:**

I did it!

Day#:

Time: _____	Glasses of Water: ☐	CALORIES	FAT	CARBS	PROTEIN	CHOLESTEROL	SODIUM	FIBER
BREAKFAST	**QTY**							
_____	___							
_____	___							
_____	___							
_____	___							
	TOTALS							

Time: _____	Glasses of Water: ☐	CALORIES	FAT	CARBS	PROTEIN	CHOLESTEROL	SODIUM	FIBER
LUNCH	**QTY**							
_____	___							
_____	___							
_____	___							
_____	___							
_____	___							
	TOTALS							

Time: _____	Glasses of Water: ☐	CALORIES	FAT	CARBS	PROTEIN	CHOLESTEROL	SODIUM	FIBER
DINNER	**QTY**							
_____	___							
_____	___							
_____	___							
_____	___							
_____	___							
_____	___							
	TOTALS							

Date: _____   Day of Week: _____

CALORIES	FAT	CARBS	PROTEIN	CHOLESTEROL	SODIUM	FIBER

Time: _____   Glasses of Water: ☐

SNACKS   **QTY**

_____   _____
_____   _____
_____   _____
_____   _____

TOTALS

Daily Totals

CALORIES	FAT	CARBS	PROTEIN	CHOLESTEROL	SODIUM	FIBER

Total Glasses of Water: ☐

Weight: _____ lbs

RATING

☺
😐
☹

EXERCISE/DAILY ACTIVITIES

Description	Time	Qty

VITAMINS/SUPPLEMENTS

Description	Time	Qty

Notes: _____
_____
_____
_____

Day #:

Time:_____	Glasses of Water: ☐	CALORIES	FAT	CARBS	PROTEIN	CHOLESTEROL	SODIUM	FIBER
BREAKFAST	**QTY**							
_____	___							
_____	___							
_____	___							
_____	___							
	TOTALS							

Time:_____	Glasses of Water: ☐	CALORIES	FAT	CARBS	PROTEIN	CHOLESTEROL	SODIUM	FIBER
LUNCH	**QTY**							
_____	___							
_____	___							
_____	___							
_____	___							
_____	___							
	TOTALS							

Time:_____	Glasses of Water: ☐	CALORIES	FAT	CARBS	PROTEIN	CHOLESTEROL	SODIUM	FIBER
DINNER	**QTY**							
_____	___							
_____	___							
_____	___							
_____	___							
_____	___							
	TOTALS							

Date: _____ Day of Week: _____

CALORIES	FAT	CARBS	PROTEIN	CHOLESTEROL	SODIUM	FIBER

Time: _____ Glasses of Water: ☐

SNACKS   **QTY**

_____   _____

_____   _____

_____   _____

_____   _____

TOTALS

Daily Totals

CALORIES	FAT	CARBS	PROTEIN	CHOLESTEROL	SODIUM	FIBER

Total Glasses of Water: ☐

Weight: _____ lbs

RATING

☺

😐

☹

EXERCISE/DAILY ACTIVITIES

Description	Time	Qty

VITAMINS/SUPPLEMENTS

Description	Time	Qty

Notes:

Day #:

Time: _____ Glasses of Water: ☐	CALORIES	FAT	CARBS	PROTEIN	CHOLESTEROL	SODIUM	FIBER
BREAKFAST QTY							
_____ ___							
_____ ___							
_____ ___							
_____ ___ TOTALS							

Time: _____ Glasses of Water: ☐	CALORIES	FAT	CARBS	PROTEIN	CHOLESTEROL	SODIUM	FIBER
LUNCH QTY							
_____ ___							
_____ ___							
_____ ___							
_____ ___							
_____ ___ TOTALS							

Time: _____ Glasses of Water: ☐	CALORIES	FAT	CARBS	PROTEIN	CHOLESTEROL	SODIUM	FIBER
DINNER QTY							
_____ ___							
_____ ___							
_____ ___							
_____ ___							
_____ ___ TOTALS							

Date: _____   Day of Week: _____

CALORIES	FAT	CARBS	PROTEIN	CHOLESTEROL	SODIUM	FIBER

Time: _____   Glasses of Water: ☐

SNACKS   **QTY**

_____   _____

_____   _____

_____   _____

_____   _____

TOTALS

Daily Totals						
CALORIES	FAT	CARBS	PROTEIN	CHOLESTEROL	SODIUM	FIBER

Total Glasses of Water: ☐

Weight: _____ lbs

RATING

☺

😐

☹

EXERCISE/DAILY ACTIVITIES

Description	Time	Qty

VITAMINS/SUPPLEMENTS

Description	Time	Qty

Notes:

Day#:

Time:_____	Glasses of Water: ☐	CALORIES	FAT	CARBS	PROTEIN	CHOLESTEROL	SODIUM	FIBER
BREAKFAST	**QTY**							
_____	___							
_____	___							
_____	___							
_____	___							
	TOTALS							

Time:_____	Glasses of Water: ☐	CALORIES	FAT	CARBS	PROTEIN	CHOLESTEROL	SODIUM	FIBER
LUNCH	**QTY**							
_____	___							
_____	___							
_____	___							
_____	___							
_____	___							
	TOTALS							

Time:_____	Glasses of Water: ☐	CALORIES	FAT	CARBS	PROTEIN	CHOLESTEROL	SODIUM	FIBER
DINNER	**QTY**							
_____	___							
_____	___							
_____	___							
_____	___							
_____	___							
	TOTALS							

14

Date: _____   Day of Week: _____

CALORIES	FAT	CARBS	PROTEIN	CHOLESTEROL	SODIUM	FIBER

Time: _____   Glasses of Water: ☐

SNACKS   **QTY**

_____   _____

_____   _____

_____   _____

_____   _____

TOTALS

Daily Totals

CALORIES	FAT	CARBS	PROTEIN	CHOLESTEROL	SODIUM	FIBER

Total Glasses of Water: ☐

Weight: _____ lbs

RATING

☺

☺

☹

EXERCISE/DAILY ACTIVITIES

Description	Time	Qty

VITAMINS/SUPPLEMENTS

Description	Time	Qty

Notes: _____

Day#: _____

Time: _____	Glasses of Water: ☐	CALORIES	FAT	CARBS	PROTEIN	CHOLESTEROL	SODIUM	FIBER
BREAKFAST	QTY							
_____	___							
_____	___							
_____	___							
_____	___							
	TOTALS							

Time: _____	Glasses of Water: ☐	CALORIES	FAT	CARBS	PROTEIN	CHOLESTEROL	SODIUM	FIBER
LUNCH	QTY							
_____	___							
_____	___							
_____	___							
_____	___							
_____	___							
	TOTALS							

Time: _____	Glasses of Water: ☐	CALORIES	FAT	CARBS	PROTEIN	CHOLESTEROL	SODIUM	FIBER
DINNER	QTY							
_____	___							
_____	___							
_____	___							
_____	___							
_____	___							
	TOTALS							

Date: _____   Day of Week: _____

CALORIES	FAT	CARBS	PROTEIN	CHOLESTEROL	SODIUM	FIBER

Time: _____   Glasses of Water: ☐

SNACKS   **QTY**

_____   _____

_____   _____

_____   _____

_____   _____

TOTALS

Daily Totals						
CALORIES	FAT	CARBS	PROTEIN	CHOLESTEROL	SODIUM	FIBER

Total Glasses of Water: ☐

Weight: _____ lbs

RATING

☺

😐

☹

EXERCISE/DAILY ACTIVITIES

Description	Time	Qty

VITAMINS/SUPPLEMENTS

Description	Time	Qty

Notes:

Day #: _____

Time: _____ Glasses of Water: ☐

	CALORIES	FAT	CARBS	PROTEIN	CHOLESTEROL	SODIUM	FIBER
BREAKFAST QTY							
_____ ___							
_____ ___							
_____ ___							
_____ ___							
TOTALS							

Time: _____ Glasses of Water: ☐

	CALORIES	FAT	CARBS	PROTEIN	CHOLESTEROL	SODIUM	FIBER
LUNCH QTY							
_____ ___							
_____ ___							
_____ ___							
_____ ___							
TOTALS							

Time: _____ Glasses of Water: ☐

	CALORIES	FAT	CARBS	PROTEIN	CHOLESTEROL	SODIUM	FIBER
DINNER QTY							
_____ ___							
_____ ___							
_____ ___							
_____ ___							
TOTALS							

Date: _____ **Day of Week:** _____

CALORIES	FAT	CARBS	PROTEIN	CHOLESTEROL	SODIUM	FIBER

Time: _____ **Glasses of Water:** ☐

SNACKS   QTY

_____ _____

_____ _____

_____ _____

_____ _____

TOTALS

Daily Totals

CALORIES	FAT	CARBS	PROTEIN	CHOLESTEROL	SODIUM	FIBER

Total Glasses of Water: ☐

Weight: _____ lbs

RATING

☺

😐

☹

EXERCISE/DAILY ACTIVITIES

Description	Time	Qty

VITAMINS/SUPPLEMENTS

Description	Time	Qty

Notes:

19

Day #: _____

Time: _____	Glasses of Water: ☐	CALORIES	FAT	CARBS	PROTEIN	CHOLESTEROL	SODIUM	FIBER
BREAKFAST	**QTY**							
_____	___							
_____	___							
_____	___							
_____	___							
	TOTALS							

Time: _____	Glasses of Water: ☐	CALORIES	FAT	CARBS	PROTEIN	CHOLESTEROL	SODIUM	FIBER
LUNCH	**QTY**							
_____	___							
_____	___							
_____	___							
_____	___							
_____	___							
	TOTALS							

Time: _____	Glasses of Water: ☐	CALORIES	FAT	CARBS	PROTEIN	CHOLESTEROL	SODIUM	FIBER
DINNER	**QTY**							
_____	___							
_____	___							
_____	___							
_____	___							
_____	___							
	TOTALS							

Date: | Day of Week:

CALORIES	FAT	CARBS	PROTEIN	CHOLESTEROL	SODIUM	FIBER

Time: _____ | Glasses of Water: ☐

SNACKS | **QTY**

_____ ___
_____ ___
_____ ___
_____ ___

TOTALS

Daily Totals

CALORIES	FAT	CARBS	PROTEIN	CHOLESTEROL	SODIUM	FIBER

Total Glasses of Water: ☐

Weight: _____ lbs

RATING

☺
😐
☹

EXERCISE/DAILY ACTIVITIES

Description	Time	Qty

VITAMINS/SUPPLEMENTS

Description	Time	Qty

Notes:

WEEKLY PROGRESS

Clothing size and change in fit:
_____

_____

_____

MEASUREMENTS:

Chest: _____

Waist: _____

Hips: _____

Thigh: _____

Weight: _____

Nutrition/Diet plan followed:

_____ %

Physical activity plan followed:

_____ %

Weekly Totals						
CALORIES	FAT	CARBS	PROTEIN	CHOLESTEROL	SODIUM	FIBER

This week's achievements: _____

_____

_____

_____

Changes and adjustments for next week: _____

_____

_____

_____

DIET TIPS

✓ Make an appointment with yourself to begin your diet.

✓ Set up a reward system for yourself that does not include food items. At the beginning of your diet, purchase gift certificates for things like movies, long-distance calls, books, new clothes. Use these as rewards.

✓ Put together your team! Perhaps your team includes your best friend to encourage and help you, a nutritionist who can assist you, your doctor for a physical exam and direction, a trainer or other exercise expert, your spouse, kids, co-workers, or others who can help and encourage you. Communicate what they can do specifically to assist you and don't be afraid to ask for help or encouragement.

Day #: _____

BREAKFAST

Time: _____ Glasses of Water: ☐

	CALORIES	FAT	CARBS	PROTEIN	CHOLESTEROL	SODIUM	FIBER
BREAKFAST — QTY							
_____ ___							
_____ ___							
_____ ___							
_____ ___							
TOTALS							

LUNCH

Time: _____ Glasses of Water: ☐

	CALORIES	FAT	CARBS	PROTEIN	CHOLESTEROL	SODIUM	FIBER
LUNCH — QTY							
_____ ___							
_____ ___							
_____ ___							
_____ ___							
TOTALS							

DINNER

Time: _____ Glasses of Water: ☐

	CALORIES	FAT	CARBS	PROTEIN	CHOLESTEROL	SODIUM	FIBER
DINNER — QTY							
_____ ___							
_____ ___							
_____ ___							
_____ ___							
TOTALS							

Date:							Day of Week:

CALORIES	FAT	CARBS	PROTEIN	CHOLESTEROL	SODIUM	FIBER

Time: _____ Glasses of Water: ▢

SNACKS   QTY

_____ ____
_____ ____
_____ ____
_____ ____

TOTALS

Daily Totals						
CALORIES	FAT	CARBS	PROTEIN	CHOLESTEROL	SODIUM	FIBER

Total Glasses of Water: ▢

Weight: _____ lbs

RATING

☺

😐

☹

EXERCISE/DAILY ACTIVITIES

Description	Time	Qty

VITAMINS/SUPPLEMENTS

Description	Time	Qty

Notes:

Day #:

Time: _____	Glasses of Water: ☐	CALORIES	FAT	CARBS	PROTEIN	CHOLESTEROL	SODIUM	FIBER
BREAKFAST	QTY							
_____	___							
_____	___							
_____	___							
_____	___							
	TOTALS							

Time: _____	Glasses of Water: ☐	CALORIES	FAT	CARBS	PROTEIN	CHOLESTEROL	SODIUM	FIBER
LUNCH	QTY							
_____	___							
_____	___							
_____	___							
_____	___							
	TOTALS							

Time: _____	Glasses of Water: ☐	CALORIES	FAT	CARBS	PROTEIN	CHOLESTEROL	SODIUM	FIBER
DINNER	QTY							
_____	___							
_____	___							
_____	___							
_____	___							
_____	___							
	TOTALS							

CALORIES	FAT	CARBS	PROTEIN	CHOLESTEROL	SODIUM	FIBER

Time: _____   Glasses of Water: ☐

SNACKS   **QTY**

_____ _____
_____ _____
_____ _____
_____ _____

TOTALS

Daily Totals

CALORIES	FAT	CARBS	PROTEIN	CHOLESTEROL	SODIUM	FIBER

Total Glasses of Water: ☐

Weight: _____ lbs

RATING

☺
😐
☹

EXERCISE/DAILY ACTIVITIES

Description	Time	Qty

VITAMINS/SUPPLEMENTS

Description	Time	Qty

Notes:

Day #: _____

Time: _____ Glasses of Water: ☐

BREAKFAST QTY

	CALORIES	FAT	CARBS	PROTEIN	CHOLESTEROL	SODIUM	FIBER
_____ ___							
_____ ___							
_____ ___							
_____ ___							
_____ ___ **TOTALS**							

Time: _____ Glasses of Water: ☐

LUNCH QTY

	CALORIES	FAT	CARBS	PROTEIN	CHOLESTEROL	SODIUM	FIBER
_____ ___							
_____ ___							
_____ ___							
_____ ___							
_____ ___							
_____ ___ **TOTALS**							

Time: _____ Glasses of Water: ☐

DINNER QTY

	CALORIES	FAT	CARBS	PROTEIN	CHOLESTEROL	SODIUM	FIBER
_____ ___							
_____ ___							
_____ ___							
_____ ___							
_____ ___ **TOTALS**							

28

Date: _____   Day of Week: _____

CALORIES	FAT	CARBS	PROTEIN	CHOLESTEROL	SODIUM	FIBER

Time: _____   Glasses of Water: ☐

SNACKS   **QTY**

_____   _____

_____   _____

_____   _____

_____   _____

TOTALS

Daily Totals

CALORIES	FAT	CARBS	PROTEIN	CHOLESTEROL	SODIUM	FIBER

Total Glasses of Water: ☐

Weight: _____ lbs

RATING

☺

😐

☹

EXERCISE/DAILY ACTIVITIES

Description	Time	Qty

VITAMINS/SUPPLEMENTS

Description	Time	Qty

Notes: _____

_____

_____

_____

Day#: _____

Time: _____	Glasses of Water: ☐	CALORIES	FAT	CARBS	PROTEIN	CHOLESTEROL	SODIUM	FIBER
BREAKFAST	**QTY**							
_____	___							
_____	___							
_____	___							
_____	___							
	TOTALS							

Time: _____	Glasses of Water: ☐	CALORIES	FAT	CARBS	PROTEIN	CHOLESTEROL	SODIUM	FIBER
LUNCH	**QTY**							
_____	___							
_____	___							
_____	___							
_____	___							
_____	___							
	TOTALS							

Time: _____	Glasses of Water: ☐	CALORIES	FAT	CARBS	PROTEIN	CHOLESTEROL	SODIUM	FIBER
DINNER	**QTY**							
_____	___							
_____	___							
_____	___							
_____	___							
_____	___							
	TOTALS							

Date: _____ **Day of Week:** _____

CALORIES	FAT	CARBS	PROTEIN	CHOLESTEROL	SODIUM	FIBER

Time: _____ **Glasses of Water:** ☐

SNACKS   QTY

_____   _____

_____   _____

_____   _____

_____   _____

TOTALS

Daily Totals

CALORIES	FAT	CARBS	PROTEIN	CHOLESTEROL	SODIUM	FIBER

Total Glasses of Water: ☐

Weight: _____ lbs

RATING

☺

😐

☹

EXERCISE/DAILY ACTIVITIES

Description	Time	Qty

VITAMINS/SUPPLEMENTS

Description	Time	Qty

Notes:

31

Day #:

Time: _____	Glasses of Water: ⬚	CALORIES	FAT	CARBS	PROTEIN	CHOLESTEROL	SODIUM	FIBER
BREAKFAST	**QTY**							
_____	___							
_____	___							
_____	___							
_____	___							
	TOTALS							

Time: _____	Glasses of Water: ⬚	CALORIES	FAT	CARBS	PROTEIN	CHOLESTEROL	SODIUM	FIBER
LUNCH	**QTY**							
_____	___							
_____	___							
_____	___							
_____	___							
	TOTALS							

Time: _____	Glasses of Water: ⬚	CALORIES	FAT	CARBS	PROTEIN	CHOLESTEROL	SODIUM	FIBER
DINNER	**QTY**							
_____	___							
_____	___							
_____	___							
_____	___							
	TOTALS							

Date:							Day of Week:

CALORIES	FAT	CARBS	PROTEIN	CHOLESTEROL	SODIUM	FIBER

Time: _____   Glasses of Water: ☐

SNACKS   QTY

_____ ____
_____ ____
_____ ____
_____ ____

TOTALS

Daily Totals

CALORIES	FAT	CARBS	PROTEIN	CHOLESTEROL	SODIUM	FIBER

Total Glasses of Water: ☐

Weight: _____ lbs

RATING
☺
😐
☹

EXERCISE/DAILY ACTIVITIES

Description	Time	Qty

VITAMINS/SUPPLEMENTS

Description	Time	Qty

Notes:

Day #:

Time: _____	Glasses of Water: ☐	CALORIES	FAT	CARBS	PROTEIN	CHOLESTEROL	SODIUM	FIBER
BREAKFAST	QTY							
_____	__							
_____	__							
_____	__							
_____	__							
	TOTALS							

Time: _____	Glasses of Water: ☐	CALORIES	FAT	CARBS	PROTEIN	CHOLESTEROL	SODIUM	FIBER
LUNCH	QTY							
_____	__							
_____	__							
_____	__							
_____	__							
_____	__							
	TOTALS							

Time: _____	Glasses of Water: ☐	CALORIES	FAT	CARBS	PROTEIN	CHOLESTEROL	SODIUM	FIBER
DINNER	QTY							
_____	__							
_____	__							
_____	__							
_____	__							
_____	__							
	TOTALS							

Date:							Day of Week:	

CALORIES	FAT	CARBS	PROTEIN	CHOLESTEROL	SODIUM	FIBER

Time: _____

Glasses of Water: ☐

SNACKS   QTY

_____ ____

_____ ____

_____ ____

_____ ____

TOTALS

Daily Totals

CALORIES	FAT	CARBS	PROTEIN	CHOLESTEROL	SODIUM	FIBER

Total Glasses of Water: ☐

Weight: _____ lbs

RATING

☺

☺/☹ (neutral)

☹

EXERCISE/DAILY ACTIVITIES

Description	Time	Qty

VITAMINS/SUPPLEMENTS

Description	Time	Qty

Notes:

Day #:

Time: _____	Glasses of Water: ▢	CALORIES	FAT	CARBS	PROTEIN	CHOLESTEROL	SODIUM	FIBER
BREAKFAST	**QTY**							
_____	____							
_____	____							
_____	____							
_____	____							
	TOTALS							

Time: _____	Glasses of Water: ▢	CALORIES	FAT	CARBS	PROTEIN	CHOLESTEROL	SODIUM	FIBER
LUNCH	**QTY**							
_____	____							
_____	____							
_____	____							
_____	____							
_____	____							
	TOTALS							

Time: _____	Glasses of Water: ▢	CALORIES	FAT	CARBS	PROTEIN	CHOLESTEROL	SODIUM	FIBER
DINNER	**QTY**							
_____	____							
_____	____							
_____	____							
_____	____							
_____	____							
	TOTALS							

Date: _____   Day of Week: _____

CALORIES	FAT	CARBS	PROTEIN	CHOLESTEROL	SODIUM	FIBER

Time: _____   Glasses of Water: ☐

SNACKS   QTY

_____	_____
_____	_____
_____	_____
_____	_____

TOTALS

Daily Totals

CALORIES	FAT	CARBS	PROTEIN	CHOLESTEROL	SODIUM	FIBER

Total Glasses of Water: ☐

Weight: _____ lbs

RATING

☺
😐
☹

EXERCISE/DAILY ACTIVITIES

Description	Time	Qty

VITAMINS/SUPPLEMENTS

Description	Time	Qty

Notes: _____

WEEKLY PROGRESS

Clothing size and change in fit:

_____

_____

MEASUREMENTS:

Chest: _____

Waist: _____

Hips: _____

Thigh: _____

Weight: _____

Nutrition/Diet plan followed:
_____%

Physical activity plan followed:
_____%

Weekly Totals						
CALORIES	FAT	CARBS	PROTEIN	CHOLESTEROL	SODIUM	FIBER

This week's achievements:

_____

_____

_____

Changes and adjustments for next week:

_____

_____

_____

_____

DIET TIPS

✓Each morning, fill a pitcher with the water you plan to drink today (at least 8 cups) and place it in the fridge. Anytime you use water, pour it from this pitcher. This includes water to make tea, coffee, or juice. Now it will be much easier to recognize when you need to increase your water intake and know when you've met your daily goal.

✓Set up a budget for new clothes to be purchased throughout your diet. Be sure to buy or borrow clothes that fit you well as you are losing weight. Compliments help you recognize your accomplishment.

✓Take it one day at a time. Renew your resolution every day. Visualize your commitment for this 24 hours and own it.

Day#:

Time: _____ Glasses of Water: ☐

BREAKFAST QTY

	CALORIES	FAT	CARBS	PROTEIN	CHOLESTEROL	SODIUM	FIBER
_____ ___							
_____ ___							
_____ ___							
_____ ___							
TOTALS							

Time: _____ Glasses of Water: ☐

LUNCH QTY

	CALORIES	FAT	CARBS	PROTEIN	CHOLESTEROL	SODIUM	FIBER
_____ ___							
_____ ___							
_____ ___							
_____ ___							
_____ ___							
TOTALS							

Time: _____ Glasses of Water: ☐

DINNER QTY

	CALORIES	FAT	CARBS	PROTEIN	CHOLESTEROL	SODIUM	FIBER
_____ ___							
_____ ___							
_____ ___							
_____ ___							
_____ ___							
TOTALS							

Date: _____   Day of Week: _____

CALORIES	FAT	CARBS	PROTEIN	CHOLESTEROL	SODIUM	FIBER

Time: _____   Glasses of Water: ☐

SNACKS   QTY

_____   _____
_____   _____
_____   _____
_____   _____

TOTALS

Daily Totals

CALORIES	FAT	CARBS	PROTEIN	CHOLESTEROL	SODIUM	FIBER

Total Glasses of Water: ☐

Weight: _____ lbs

RATING

☺
😐
☹

EXERCISE/DAILY ACTIVITIES

Description	Time	Qty

VITAMINS/SUPPLEMENTS

Description	Time	Qty

Notes:

41

Day #: _____

Time: _____ Glasses of Water: ▢	CALORIES	FAT	CARBS	PROTEIN	CHOLESTEROL	SODIUM	FIBER
BREAKFAST QTY							
_____ ___							
_____ ___							
_____ ___							
_____ ___							
TOTALS							

Time: _____ Glasses of Water: ▢	CALORIES	FAT	CARBS	PROTEIN	CHOLESTEROL	SODIUM	FIBER
LUNCH QTY							
_____ ___							
_____ ___							
_____ ___							
_____ ___							
_____ ___							
TOTALS							

Time: _____ Glasses of Water: ▢	CALORIES	FAT	CARBS	PROTEIN	CHOLESTEROL	SODIUM	FIBER
DINNER QTY							
_____ ___							
_____ ___							
_____ ___							
_____ ___							
_____ ___							
TOTALS							

Date:							Day of Week:

CALORIES	FAT	CARBS	PROTEIN	CHOLESTEROL	SODIUM	FIBER

Time: _____ Glasses of Water: ☐

SNACKS   **QTY**

_____ _____

_____ _____

_____ _____

_____ _____

TOTALS

Daily Totals

CALORIES	FAT	CARBS	PROTEIN	CHOLESTEROL	SODIUM	FIBER

Total Glasses of Water: ☐

Weight: _____ lbs

RATING

☺

😐

☹

EXERCISE/DAILY ACTIVITIES

Description	Time	Qty

VITAMINS/SUPPLEMENTS

Description	Time	Qty

Notes:

Day#:

Time: _____	Glasses of Water: ☐	CALORIES	FAT	CARBS	PROTEIN	CHOLESTEROL	SODIUM	FIBER
BREAKFAST	QTY							
_____	____							
_____	____							
_____	____							
_____	____							
	TOTALS							

Time: _____	Glasses of Water: ☐	CALORIES	FAT	CARBS	PROTEIN	CHOLESTEROL	SODIUM	FIBER
LUNCH	QTY							
_____	____							
_____	____							
_____	____							
_____	____							
_____	____							
	TOTALS							

Time: _____	Glasses of Water: ☐	CALORIES	FAT	CARBS	PROTEIN	CHOLESTEROL	SODIUM	FIBER
DINNER	QTY							
_____	____							
_____	____							
_____	____							
_____	____							
_____	____							
	TOTALS							

44

Date:							Day of Week:

CALORIES	FAT	CARBS	PROTEIN	CHOLESTEROL	SODIUM	FIBER

Time:_____ Glasses of Water: ☐

SNACKS   QTY

_____ ____
_____ ____
_____ ____
_____ ____

TOTALS

Daily Totals

CALORIES	FAT	CARBS	PROTEIN	CHOLESTEROL	SODIUM	FIBER

Total Glasses of Water: ☐

Weight: _____ lbs

RATING

☺
😐
☹

EXERCISE/DAILY ACTIVITIES

Description	Time	Qty

VITAMINS/SUPPLEMENTS

Description	Time	Qty

Notes:

Day#:

Time:_____ Glasses of Water: ☐

BREAKFAST   QTY

	CALORIES	FAT	CARBS	PROTEIN	CHOLESTEROL	SODIUM	FIBER
_____ ____							
_____ ____							
_____ ____							
_____ ____							
TOTALS							

Time:_____ Glasses of Water: ☐

LUNCH   QTY

	CALORIES	FAT	CARBS	PROTEIN	CHOLESTEROL	SODIUM	FIBER
_____ ____							
_____ ____							
_____ ____							
_____ ____							
_____ ____							
TOTALS							

Time:_____ Glasses of Water: ☐

DINNER   QTY

	CALORIES	FAT	CARBS	PROTEIN	CHOLESTEROL	SODIUM	FIBER
_____ ____							
_____ ____							
_____ ____							
_____ ____							
_____ ____							
TOTALS							

Date:	Day of Week:

CALORIES	FAT	CARBS	PROTEIN	CHOLESTEROL	SODIUM	FIBER

Time: _____ Glasses of Water: ☐

SNACKS   QTY

_____ ___
_____ ___
_____ ___
_____ ___

TOTALS

Daily Totals

CALORIES	FAT	CARBS	PROTEIN	CHOLESTEROL	SODIUM	FIBER

Total Glasses of Water: ☐

Weight: _____ lbs

RATING

☺
😐
☹

EXERCISE/DAILY ACTIVITIES

Description	Time	Qty

VITAMINS/SUPPLEMENTS

Description	Time	Qty

Notes:

47

Day#:

Time: _____	Glasses of Water:	CALORIES	FAT	CARBS	PROTEIN	CHOLESTEROL	SODIUM	FIBER
BREAKFAST	QTY							
_____	___							
_____	___							
_____	___							
_____	___							
	TOTALS							

Time: _____	Glasses of Water:	CALORIES	FAT	CARBS	PROTEIN	CHOLESTEROL	SODIUM	FIBER
LUNCH	QTY							
_____	___							
_____	___							
_____	___							
_____	___							
_____	___							
	TOTALS							

Time: _____	Glasses of Water:	CALORIES	FAT	CARBS	PROTEIN	CHOLESTEROL	SODIUM	FIBER
DINNER	QTY							
_____	___							
_____	___							
_____	___							
_____	___							
_____	___							
	TOTALS							

Date:

Day of Week:

CALORIES	FAT	CARBS	PROTEIN	CHOLESTEROL	SODIUM	FIBER

Time: _____

Glasses of Water: ☐

SNACKS	**QTY**
_____	_____
_____	_____
_____	_____
_____	_____

TOTALS

Daily Totals

CALORIES	FAT	CARBS	PROTEIN	CHOLESTEROL	SODIUM	FIBER

Total Glasses of Water: ☐

Weight: _____ lbs

RATING

☺

😐

☹

EXERCISE/DAILY ACTIVITIES

Description	Time	Qty

VITAMINS/SUPPLEMENTS

Description	Time	Qty

Notes:

Day#:

BREAKFAST

Time: _____	Glasses of Water:							
BREAKFAST	**QTY**	CALORIES	FAT	CARBS	PROTEIN	CHOLESTEROL	SODIUM	FIBER
_____	____							
_____	____							
_____	____							
_____	**TOTALS**							

LUNCH

Time: _____	Glasses of Water:							
LUNCH	**QTY**	CALORIES	FAT	CARBS	PROTEIN	CHOLESTEROL	SODIUM	FIBER
_____	____							
_____	____							
_____	____							
_____	____							
_____	**TOTALS**							

DINNER

Time: _____	Glasses of Water:							
DINNER	**QTY**	CALORIES	FAT	CARBS	PROTEIN	CHOLESTEROL	SODIUM	FIBER
_____	____							
_____	____							
_____	____							
_____	____							
_____	**TOTALS**							

Date:							Day of Week:	

CALORIES	FAT	CARBS	PROTEIN	CHOLESTEROL	SODIUM	FIBER

Time:_____ Glasses of Water: ⬜

SNACKS   QTY

_____ ____
_____ ____
_____ ____
_____ ____

TOTALS

Daily Totals

CALORIES	FAT	CARBS	PROTEIN	CHOLESTEROL	SODIUM	FIBER

Total Glasses of Water: ⬜

Weight: _____ lbs

RATING

☺

😐

☹

EXERCISE/DAILY ACTIVITIES

Description	Time	Qty

VITAMINS/SUPPLEMENTS

Description	Time	Qty

Notes:

Day#:

	CALORIES	FAT	CARBS	PROTEIN	CHOLESTEROL	SODIUM	FIBER

Time:_____ Glasses of Water: ☐

BREAKFAST QTY

___ ___							
___ ___							
___ ___							
___ ___							
TOTALS							

Time:_____ Glasses of Water: ☐

LUNCH QTY

	CALORIES	FAT	CARBS	PROTEIN	CHOLESTEROL	SODIUM	FIBER
___ ___							
___ ___							
___ ___							
___ ___							
___ ___							
TOTALS							

Time:_____ Glasses of Water: ☐

DINNER QTY

	CALORIES	FAT	CARBS	PROTEIN	CHOLESTEROL	SODIUM	FIBER
___ ___							
___ ___							
___ ___							
___ ___							
___ ___							
TOTALS							

Date: | Day of Week:

CALORIES	FAT	CARBS	PROTEIN	CHOLESTEROL	SODIUM	FIBER

Time:_____ Glasses of Water: ☐

SNACKS | QTY

_____ _____
_____ _____
_____ _____
_____ _____

TOTALS

Daily Totals

CALORIES	FAT	CARBS	PROTEIN	CHOLESTEROL	SODIUM	FIBER

Total Glasses of Water: ☐

Weight: _____ lbs

RATING

☺
😐
☹

EXERCISE/DAILY ACTIVITIES

Description	Time	Qty

VITAMINS/SUPPLEMENTS

Description	Time	Qty

Notes:

53

WEEKLY PROGRESS

Clothing size and change in fit: _____

_____

_____

MEASUREMENTS:

Chest: _____

Waist: _____

Hips: _____

Thigh: _____

Weight: _____

Nutrition/Diet plan followed:

_____ %

Physical activity plan followed:

_____ %

Weekly Totals						
CALORIES	FAT	CARBS	PROTEIN	CHOLESTEROL	SODIUM	FIBER

This week's achievements: _____

_____

_____

_____

Changes and adjustments for next week: _____

_____

_____

_____

DIET TIPS

✓Give up eating in the car or on the run. This will eliminate a lot of poor eating choices.

✓Identify the "treat" foods on your diet and look forward to them, replacing foods restricted from your diet.

✓Plan a work session each week to prepare special food items on your diet and have them ready to eat when you need or want a snack.

✓Rearrange your refrigerator. If family members eat foods not included on your diet, place those foods at the bottom of the fridge. Move the foods you need to the top shelf so they are what you see when you open the door.

Day #:

BREAKFAST	QTY	CALORIES	FAT	CARBS	PROTEIN	CHOLESTEROL	SODIUM	FIBER
Time: _____	Glasses of Water:							
_____	___							
_____	___							
_____	___							
_____	___							
	TOTALS							

LUNCH	QTY	CALORIES	FAT	CARBS	PROTEIN	CHOLESTEROL	SODIUM	FIBER
Time: _____	Glasses of Water:							
_____	___							
_____	___							
_____	___							
_____	___							
_____	___							
	TOTALS							

DINNER	QTY	CALORIES	FAT	CARBS	PROTEIN	CHOLESTEROL	SODIUM	FIBER
Time: _____	Glasses of Water:							
_____	___							
_____	___							
_____	___							
_____	___							
_____	___							
	TOTALS							

Date:							Day of Week:	

CALORIES	FAT	CARBS	PROTEIN	CHOLESTEROL	SODIUM	FIBER

Time:_____

Glasses of Water: ☐

SNACKS   QTY

_____ ____

_____ ____

_____ ____

_____ ____

TOTALS

Daily Totals

CALORIES	FAT	CARBS	PROTEIN	CHOLESTEROL	SODIUM	FIBER

Total Glasses of Water: ☐

RATING

☺

😐

☹

Weight: _____ lbs

EXERCISE/DAILY ACTIVITIES

Description	Time	Qty

VITAMINS/SUPPLEMENTS

Description	Time	Qty

Notes:

Day#:

BREAKFAST

Time: _____   Glasses of Water: ⬚

BREAKFAST	QTY	CALORIES	FAT	CARBS	PROTEIN	CHOLESTEROL	SODIUM	FIBER
_____	___							
_____	___							
_____	___							
_____	___							
TOTALS								

LUNCH

Time: _____   Glasses of Water: ⬚

LUNCH	QTY	CALORIES	FAT	CARBS	PROTEIN	CHOLESTEROL	SODIUM	FIBER
_____	___							
_____	___							
_____	___							
_____	___							
_____	___							
TOTALS								

DINNER

Time: _____   Glasses of Water: ⬚

DINNER	QTY	CALORIES	FAT	CARBS	PROTEIN	CHOLESTEROL	SODIUM	FIBER
_____	___							
_____	___							
_____	___							
_____	___							
_____	___							
TOTALS								

Date: _____   Day of Week: _____

CALORIES	FAT	CARBS	PROTEIN	CHOLESTEROL	SODIUM	FIBER

Time: _____   Glasses of Water: ☐

SNACKS   **QTY**

_____   ____

_____   ____

_____   ____

_____   ____

TOTALS

Daily Totals

CALORIES	FAT	CARBS	PROTEIN	CHOLESTEROL	SODIUM	FIBER

Total Glasses of Water: ☐

Weight: _____ lbs

RATING

☺
😐
☹

EXERCISE/DAILY ACTIVITIES

Description	Time	Qty

VITAMINS/SUPPLEMENTS

Description	Time	Qty

Notes:

Day#:

Time: _____ Glasses of Water: ☐	CALORIES	FAT	CARBS	PROTEIN	CHOLESTEROL	SODIUM	FIBER
BREAKFAST QTY							
_____ ___							
_____ ___							
_____ ___							
_____ ___							
TOTALS							

Time: _____ Glasses of Water: ☐	CALORIES	FAT	CARBS	PROTEIN	CHOLESTEROL	SODIUM	FIBER
LUNCH QTY							
_____ ___							
_____ ___							
_____ ___							
_____ ___							
_____ ___							
TOTALS							

Time: _____ Glasses of Water: ☐	CALORIES	FAT	CARBS	PROTEIN	CHOLESTEROL	SODIUM	FIBER
DINNER QTY							
_____ ___							
_____ ___							
_____ ___							
_____ ___							
_____ ___							
TOTALS							

Date: _____   Day of Week: _____

CALORIES	FAT	CARBS	PROTEIN	CHOLESTEROL	SODIUM	FIBER

Time: _____   Glasses of Water: ☐

SNACKS   **QTY**

_____   _____
_____   _____
_____   _____

TOTALS

Daily Totals

CALORIES	FAT	CARBS	PROTEIN	CHOLESTEROL	SODIUM	FIBER

Total Glasses of Water: ☐

Weight: _____ lbs

RATING

☺
😐
☹

EXERCISE/DAILY ACTIVITIES

Description	Time	Qty

VITAMINS/SUPPLEMENTS

Description	Time	Qty

Notes: _____

_____

_____

Day #: _____

Time: _____	Glasses of Water: ☐	CALORIES	FAT	CARBS	PROTEIN	CHOLESTEROL	SODIUM	FIBER
BREAKFAST	**QTY**							
_____	___							
_____	___							
_____	___							
_____	___							
	TOTALS							

Time: _____	Glasses of Water: ☐	CALORIES	FAT	CARBS	PROTEIN	CHOLESTEROL	SODIUM	FIBER
LUNCH	**QTY**							
_____	___							
_____	___							
_____	___							
_____	___							
_____	___							
	TOTALS							

Time: _____	Glasses of Water: ☐	CALORIES	FAT	CARBS	PROTEIN	CHOLESTEROL	SODIUM	FIBER
DINNER	**QTY**							
_____	___							
_____	___							
_____	___							
_____	___							
	TOTALS							

Date: _____   Day of Week: _____

CALORIES	FAT	CARBS	PROTEIN	CHOLESTEROL	SODIUM	FIBER

Time: _____   Glasses of Water: ☐

SNACKS   QTY

_____   _____
_____   _____
_____   _____
_____   _____

TOTALS

Daily Totals

CALORIES	FAT	CARBS	PROTEIN	CHOLESTEROL	SODIUM	FIBER

Total Glasses of Water: ☐

RATING

☺
😐
☹

Weight: _____ lbs

EXERCISE/DAILY ACTIVITIES

Description	Time	Qty

VITAMINS/SUPPLEMENTS

Description	Time	Qty

Notes: _____
_____
_____
_____

Day #:

Time: _____	Glasses of Water: ☐	CALORIES	FAT	CARBS	PROTEIN	CHOLESTEROL	SODIUM	FIBER
BREAKFAST	**QTY**							
_____	___							
_____	___							
_____	___							
_____	___							
	TOTALS							

Time: _____	Glasses of Water: ☐	CALORIES	FAT	CARBS	PROTEIN	CHOLESTEROL	SODIUM	FIBER
LUNCH	**QTY**							
_____	___							
_____	___							
_____	___							
_____	___							
_____	___							
	TOTALS							

Time: _____	Glasses of Water: ☐	CALORIES	FAT	CARBS	PROTEIN	CHOLESTEROL	SODIUM	FIBER
DINNER	**QTY**							
_____	___							
_____	___							
_____	___							
_____	___							
_____	___							
	TOTALS							

Date: _____

Day of Week: _____

CALORIES	FAT	CARBS	PROTEIN	CHOLESTEROL	SODIUM	FIBER

Time: _____

Glasses of Water: ☐

SNACKS   **QTY**

_____ ____

_____ ____

_____ ____

_____ ____

TOTALS

Daily Totals

CALORIES	FAT	CARBS	PROTEIN	CHOLESTEROL	SODIUM	FIBER

Total Glasses of Water: ☐

Weight: _____ lbs

RATING

☺

😐

☹

EXERCISE/DAILY ACTIVITIES

Description	Time	Qty

VITAMINS/SUPPLEMENTS

Description	Time	Qty

Notes:

Day #:

Time: _____	Glasses of Water: ☐							
BREAKFAST	**QTY**	CALORIES	FAT	CARBS	PROTEIN	CHOLESTEROL	SODIUM	FIBER
_____	____							
_____	____							
_____	____							
_____	____							
	TOTALS							

Time: _____	Glasses of Water: ☐							
LUNCH	**QTY**	CALORIES	FAT	CARBS	PROTEIN	CHOLESTEROL	SODIUM	FIBER
_____	____							
_____	____							
_____	____							
_____	____							
_____	____							
	TOTALS							

Time: _____	Glasses of Water: ☐							
DINNER	**QTY**	CALORIES	FAT	CARBS	PROTEIN	CHOLESTEROL	SODIUM	FIBER
_____	____							
_____	____							
_____	____							
_____	____							
_____	____							
	TOTALS							

Date: _____ **Day of Week:** _____

CALORIES	FAT	CARBS	PROTEIN	CHOLESTEROL	SODIUM	FIBER

Time: _____ **Glasses of Water:** ☐

SNACKS   QTY

_____ _____

_____ _____

_____ _____

_____ _____

TOTALS

Daily Totals

CALORIES	FAT	CARBS	PROTEIN	CHOLESTEROL	SODIUM	FIBER

Total Glasses of Water: ☐

Weight: _____ lbs

RATING

☺

😐

☹

EXERCISE/DAILY ACTIVITIES

Description	Time	Qty

VITAMINS/SUPPLEMENTS

Description	Time	Qty

Notes:

Day #: _____

Time: _____	Glasses of Water: ☐	CALORIES	FAT	CARBS	PROTEIN	CHOLESTEROL	SODIUM	FIBER
BREAKFAST	QTY							
_____	___							
_____	___							
_____	___							
_____	___							
	TOTALS							

Time: _____	Glasses of Water: ☐	CALORIES	FAT	CARBS	PROTEIN	CHOLESTEROL	SODIUM	FIBER
LUNCH	QTY							
_____	___							
_____	___							
_____	___							
_____	___							
_____	___							
	TOTALS							

Time: _____	Glasses of Water: ☐	CALORIES	FAT	CARBS	PROTEIN	CHOLESTEROL	SODIUM	FIBER
DINNER	QTY							
_____	___							
_____	___							
_____	___							
_____	___							
_____	___							
	TOTALS							

| Date: | | | | | | | Day of Week: |

CALORIES	FAT	CARBS	PROTEIN	CHOLESTEROL	SODIUM	FIBER

Time: _____   Glasses of Water: ☐

SNACKS   **QTY**

_____   _____
_____   _____
_____   _____
_____   _____

TOTALS

Daily Totals

CALORIES	FAT	CARBS	PROTEIN	CHOLESTEROL	SODIUM	FIBER

Total Glasses of Water: ☐

Weight: _____ lbs

RATING

☺

😐

☹

EXERCISE/DAILY ACTIVITIES

Description	Time	Qty

VITAMINS/SUPPLEMENTS

Description	Time	Qty

Notes:

69

WEEKLY PROGRESS

Clothing size and change in fit: _____

_____

_____

MEASUREMENTS:

Chest: _____

Waist: _____

Hips: _____

Thigh: _____

Weight: _____

Nutrition/Diet plan followed:
_____ %

Physical activity plan followed:
_____ %

Weekly Totals						
CALORIES	FAT	CARBS	PROTEIN	CHOLESTEROL	SODIUM	FIBER

This week's achievements: _____

_____

_____

_____

Changes and adjustments for next week: _____

_____

_____

_____

DIET TIPS

✓Eat smaller, more frequent meals. Eat larger meals earlier in the day. Don't skip meals and don't let yourself get hungry.

✓Make yourself an emergency kit. Put in it whatever will encourage you. Ask your friends to write you notes of encouragement and seal them up. Include inspirational quotes and verses. Perhaps pictures of yourself at your desired weight. Even a swimsuit in the size you plan to reach. Whatever will keep you motivated.

✓Take time to enjoy the foods you eat. Slow down and really taste the food.

✓When traveling, pack a food bag with items on your diet. Always assume that appropriate foods will not be available and you will want to have something available when others are eating.

Day#:

Time:	Glasses of Water: ☐	CALORIES	FAT	CARBS	PROTEIN	CHOLESTEROL	SODIUM	FIBER
BREAKFAST	**QTY**							
_____	___							
_____	___							
_____	___							
_____	___							
_____	**TOTALS**							

Time:	Glasses of Water: ☐	CALORIES	FAT	CARBS	PROTEIN	CHOLESTEROL	SODIUM	FIBER
LUNCH	**QTY**							
_____	___							
_____	___							
_____	___							
_____	___							
_____	___							
_____	**TOTALS**							

Time:	Glasses of Water: ☐	CALORIES	FAT	CARBS	PROTEIN	CHOLESTEROL	SODIUM	FIBER
DINNER	**QTY**							
_____	___							
_____	___							
_____	___							
_____	___							
_____	___							
_____	**TOTALS**							

Date: _____   Day of Week: _____

CALORIES	FAT	CARBS	PROTEIN	CHOLESTEROL	SODIUM	FIBER

Time: _____   Glasses of Water: ☐

SNACKS   **QTY**

_____   ____

_____   ____

_____   ____

_____   ____

TOTALS

Daily Totals

CALORIES	FAT	CARBS	PROTEIN	CHOLESTEROL	SODIUM	FIBER

Total Glasses of Water: ☐

Weight: _____ lbs

RATING

☺

😐

☹

EXERCISE/DAILY ACTIVITIES

Description	Time	Qty

VITAMINS/SUPPLEMENTS

Description	Time	Qty

Notes:

Day#:

Time:_____ Glasses of Water: ☐							
BREAKFAST	**QTY**	CALORIES	FAT	CARBS	PROTEIN	CHOLESTEROL	SODIUM	FIBER

		CALORIES	FAT	CARBS	PROTEIN	CHOLESTEROL	SODIUM	FIBER
_____	___							
_____	___							
_____	___							
_____	___							
	TOTALS							

		CALORIES	FAT	CARBS	PROTEIN	CHOLESTEROL	SODIUM	FIBER
Time:_____ Glasses of Water: ☐								
LUNCH	**QTY**							
_____	___							
_____	___							
_____	___							
_____	___							
_____	___							
	TOTALS							

		CALORIES	FAT	CARBS	PROTEIN	CHOLESTEROL	SODIUM	FIBER
Time:_____ Glasses of Water: ☐								
DINNER	**QTY**							
_____	___							
_____	___							
_____	___							
_____	___							
_____	___							
	TOTALS							

Date: | Day of Week:

CALORIES	FAT	CARBS	PROTEIN	CHOLESTEROL	SODIUM	FIBER

Time: _____ | Glasses of Water: ☐

SNACKS | QTY

_____ ____

_____ ____

_____ ____

_____ ____

TOTALS

Daily Totals

CALORIES	FAT	CARBS	PROTEIN	CHOLESTEROL	SODIUM	FIBER

Total Glasses of Water: ☐

Weight: _____ lbs

RATING

☺

😐

☹

EXERCISE/DAILY ACTIVITIES

Description	Time	Qty

VITAMINS/SUPPLEMENTS

Description	Time	Qty

Notes:

Day#: _____

Time: _____	Glasses of Water: ☐							
BREAKFAST	**QTY**	CALORIES	FAT	CARBS	PROTEIN	CHOLESTEROL	SODIUM	FIBER
_____	___							
_____	___							
_____	___							
_____	___							
	TOTALS							

Time: _____	Glasses of Water: ☐							
LUNCH	**QTY**	CALORIES	FAT	CARBS	PROTEIN	CHOLESTEROL	SODIUM	FIBER
_____	___							
_____	___							
_____	___							
_____	___							
_____	___							
	TOTALS							

Time: _____	Glasses of Water: ☐							
DINNER	**QTY**	CALORIES	FAT	CARBS	PROTEIN	CHOLESTEROL	SODIUM	FIBER
_____	___							
_____	___							
_____	___							
_____	___							
_____	___							
	TOTALS							

Date: _____ Day of Week: _____

CALORIES	FAT	CARBS	PROTEIN	CHOLESTEROL	SODIUM	FIBER

Time: _____   Glasses of Water: ☐

SNACKS   QTY

_____ ___

_____ ___

_____ ___

_____ ___

TOTALS

Daily Totals

CALORIES	FAT	CARBS	PROTEIN	CHOLESTEROL	SODIUM	FIBER

Total Glasses of Water: ☐

RATING

☺

😐

☹

Weight: _____ lbs

EXERCISE/DAILY ACTIVITIES

Description	Time	Qty

VITAMINS/SUPPLEMENTS

Description	Time	Qty

Notes:

Day#:

BREAKFAST

Time:_____ Glasses of Water: ☐

BREAKFAST	QTY	CALORIES	FAT	CARBS	PROTEIN	CHOLESTEROL	SODIUM	FIBER
_____	___							
_____	___							
_____	___							
_____	TOTALS							

LUNCH

Time:_____ Glasses of Water: ☐

LUNCH	QTY	CALORIES	FAT	CARBS	PROTEIN	CHOLESTEROL	SODIUM	FIBER
_____	___							
_____	___							
_____	___							
_____	___							
_____	TOTALS							

DINNER

Time:_____ Glasses of Water: ☐

DINNER	QTY	CALORIES	FAT	CARBS	PROTEIN	CHOLESTEROL	SODIUM	FIBER
_____	___							
_____	___							
_____	___							
_____	___							
_____	TOTALS							

CALORIES	FAT	CARBS	PROTEIN	CHOLESTEROL	SODIUM	FIBER

Date: **Day of Week:**

Time: _____ **Glasses of Water:**

SNACKS

SNACKS	QTY
TOTALS	

Daily Totals

CALORIES	FAT	CARBS	PROTEIN	CHOLESTEROL	SODIUM	FIBER

Total Glasses of Water:

RATING

☺

☹

😐

☹

Weight: _____ *lbs*

EXERCISE/DAILY ACTIVITIES

Description	Time	Qty

VITAMINS/SUPPLEMENTS

Description	Time	Qty

Notes:

Day #:

Time:	Glasses of Water:	CALORIES	FAT	CARBS	PROTEIN	CHOLESTEROL	SODIUM	FIBER
BREAKFAST	**QTY**							
_____	_____							
_____	_____							
_____	_____							
_____	_____							
	TOTALS							

Time:	Glasses of Water:	CALORIES	FAT	CARBS	PROTEIN	CHOLESTEROL	SODIUM	FIBER
LUNCH	**QTY**							
_____	_____							
_____	_____							
_____	_____							
_____	_____							
_____	_____							
	TOTALS							

Time:	Glasses of Water:	CALORIES	FAT	CARBS	PROTEIN	CHOLESTEROL	SODIUM	FIBER
DINNER	**QTY**							
_____	_____							
_____	_____							
_____	_____							
_____	_____							
_____	_____							
	TOTALS							

Date:							Day of Week:

CALORIES	FAT	CARBS	PROTEIN	CHOLESTEROL	SODIUM	FIBER

Time: _____ Glasses of Water: ☐

SNACKS   QTY

_____ _____
_____ _____
_____ _____
_____ _____

TOTALS

Daily Totals						
CALORIES	FAT	CARBS	PROTEIN	CHOLESTEROL	SODIUM	FIBER

Total Glasses of Water: ☐

Weight: _____ lbs

RATING

☺

😐

☹

EXERCISE/DAILY ACTIVITIES

Description	Time	Qty

VITAMINS/SUPPLEMENTS

Description	Time	Qty

Notes:

Day#:

Time:	Glasses of Water:	CALORIES	FAT	CARBS	PROTEIN	CHOLESTEROL	SODIUM	FIBER
BREAKFAST	QTY							
_____	___							
_____	___							
_____	___							
_____	___							
	TOTALS							

Time:	Glasses of Water:	CALORIES	FAT	CARBS	PROTEIN	CHOLESTEROL	SODIUM	FIBER
LUNCH	QTY							
_____	___							
_____	___							
_____	___							
_____	___							
_____	___							
	TOTALS							

Time:	Glasses of Water:	CALORIES	FAT	CARBS	PROTEIN	CHOLESTEROL	SODIUM	FIBER
DINNER	QTY							
_____	___							
_____	___							
_____	___							
_____	___							
_____	___							
	TOTALS							

Date: _____   Day of Week: _____

CALORIES	FAT	CARBS	PROTEIN	CHOLESTEROL	SODIUM	FIBER

Time: _____   Glasses of Water: ☐

SNACKS   **QTY**

_____   _____

_____   _____

_____   _____

_____   _____

TOTALS

Daily Totals

CALORIES	FAT	CARBS	PROTEIN	CHOLESTEROL	SODIUM	FIBER

Total Glasses of Water: ☐

Weight: _____ lbs

RATING

☺

😐

☹

EXERCISE/DAILY ACTIVITIES

Description	Time	Qty

VITAMINS/SUPPLEMENTS

Description	Time	Qty

Notes:

Day #:

Time: _____ Glasses of Water: ☐

BREAKFAST | QTY

	CALORIES	FAT	CARBS	PROTEIN	CHOLESTEROL	SODIUM	FIBER
_____							
_____							
_____							
_____							
TOTALS							

Time: _____ Glasses of Water: ☐

LUNCH | QTY

	CALORIES	FAT	CARBS	PROTEIN	CHOLESTEROL	SODIUM	FIBER
_____							
_____							
_____							
_____							
_____							
TOTALS							

Time: _____ Glasses of Water: ☐

DINNER | QTY

	CALORIES	FAT	CARBS	PROTEIN	CHOLESTEROL	SODIUM	FIBER
_____							
_____							
_____							
_____							
_____							
TOTALS							

Date:							Day of Week:

CALORIES	FAT	CARBS	PROTEIN	CHOLESTEROL	SODIUM	FIBER

Time: _____   Glasses of Water: ☐

SNACKS   **QTY**

_____ _____
_____ _____
_____ _____
_____ _____

TOTALS

Daily Totals

CALORIES	FAT	CARBS	PROTEIN	CHOLESTEROL	SODIUM	FIBER

Total Glasses of Water: ☐

RATING
☺
😐
☹

Weight: _____ *lbs*

EXERCISE/DAILY ACTIVITIES

Description	Time	Qty

VITAMINS/SUPPLEMENTS

Description	Time	Qty

Notes:

WEEKLY PROGRESS

Clothing size and change in fit: _____

_____

_____

MEASUREMENTS:

Chest: _____

Waist: _____

Hips: _____

Thigh: _____

Weight: _____

Nutrition/Diet plan followed:

_____ %

Physical activity plan followed:

_____ %

	Weekly Totals					
CALORIES	FAT	CARBS	PROTEIN	CHOLESTEROL	SODIUM	FIBER

This week's achievements: _____

_____

_____

_____

Changes and adjustments for next week: _____

_____

_____

_____

DIET TIPS

✓ Consider giving up one television program daily for a half hour of exercise. Trade an indoor, less active chore for an outdoor, more active chore.

✓ Make a shopping list for the grocery store. Think of yourself as a diet strategist and your menu plan and shopping list become indispensable tools.

✓ Rent workout videos. Introduce yourself to a variety of workouts and purchase one you like.

✓ Schedule business meetings in the office rather than at restaurants.

✓ Give attention to food texture. When planning meals and snacks, remember to include food textures you desire.

Day #: _____

Time: _____	Glasses of Water: ☐							
BREAKFAST	**QTY**	CALORIES	FAT	CARBS	PROTEIN	CHOLESTEROL	SODIUM	FIBER
_____	____							
_____	____							
_____	____							
_____	____							
	TOTALS							

Time: _____	Glasses of Water: ☐							
LUNCH	**QTY**	CALORIES	FAT	CARBS	PROTEIN	CHOLESTEROL	SODIUM	FIBER
_____	____							
_____	____							
_____	____							
_____	____							
_____	____							
	TOTALS							

Time: _____	Glasses of Water: ☐							
DINNER	**QTY**	CALORIES	FAT	CARBS	PROTEIN	CHOLESTEROL	SODIUM	FIBER
_____	____							
_____	____							
_____	____							
_____	____							
_____	____							
	TOTALS							

CALORIES	FAT	CARBS	PROTEIN	CHOLESTEROL	SODIUM	FIBER

Date: _____

Day of Week: _____

Time: _____   Glasses of Water: ☐

SNACKS   QTY

_____   ____
_____   ____
_____   ____
_____   ____

TOTALS

Daily Totals

CALORIES	FAT	CARBS	PROTEIN	CHOLESTEROL	SODIUM	FIBER

Total Glasses of Water: ☐

Weight: _____ lbs

RATING

☺
😐
☹

EXERCISE/DAILY ACTIVITIES

Description	Time	Qty

VITAMINS/SUPPLEMENTS

Description	Time	Qty

Notes:
_____
_____
_____

Day #:

BREAKFAST

Time: _____ Glasses of Water: ⬜

	QTY	CALORIES	FAT	CARBS	PROTEIN	CHOLESTEROL	SODIUM	FIBER
_____	___							
_____	___							
_____	___							
_____	___							
	TOTALS							

LUNCH

Time: _____ Glasses of Water: ⬜

	QTY	CALORIES	FAT	CARBS	PROTEIN	CHOLESTEROL	SODIUM	FIBER
_____	___							
_____	___							
_____	___							
_____	___							
_____	___							
	TOTALS							

DINNER

Time: _____ Glasses of Water: ⬜

	QTY	CALORIES	FAT	CARBS	PROTEIN	CHOLESTEROL	SODIUM	FIBER
_____	___							
_____	___							
_____	___							
_____	___							
_____	___							
	TOTALS							

Date:							Day of Week:

CALORIES	FAT	CARBS	PROTEIN	CHOLESTEROL	SODIUM	FIBER

Time: _____   Glasses of Water: ☐

SNACKS   QTY

_____	____
_____	____
_____	____
_____	____

TOTALS

Daily Totals

CALORIES	FAT	CARBS	PROTEIN	CHOLESTEROL	SODIUM	FIBER

Total Glasses of Water: ☐

Weight: _____ lbs

RATING

☺
😐
☹

EXERCISE/DAILY ACTIVITIES

Description	Time	Qty

VITAMINS/SUPPLEMENTS

Description	Time	Qty

Notes:

Day#: _____

BREAKFAST	QTY	CALORIES	FAT	CARBS	PROTEIN	CHOLESTEROL	SODIUM	FIBER
Time: _____ Glasses of Water:								
_____	____							
_____	____							
_____	____							
_____	____							
TOTALS								

LUNCH	QTY	CALORIES	FAT	CARBS	PROTEIN	CHOLESTEROL	SODIUM	FIBER
Time: _____ Glasses of Water:								
_____	____							
_____	____							
_____	____							
_____	____							
_____	____							
TOTALS								

DINNER	QTY	CALORIES	FAT	CARBS	PROTEIN	CHOLESTEROL	SODIUM	FIBER
Time: _____ Glasses of Water:								
_____	____							
_____	____							
_____	____							
_____	____							
_____	____							
TOTALS								

| Date: | | | | | | | Day of Week: |

CALORIES	FAT	CARBS	PROTEIN	CHOLESTEROL	SODIUM	FIBER

Time: _____ Glasses of Water: ☐

SNACKS   QTY

_____ _____

_____ _____

_____ _____

_____ _____

TOTALS

Daily Totals

CALORIES	FAT	CARBS	PROTEIN	CHOLESTEROL	SODIUM	FIBER

Total Glasses of Water: ☐

Weight: _____ lbs

RATING

☺

😐

☹

EXERCISE/DAILY ACTIVITIES

Description	Time	Qty

VITAMINS/SUPPLEMENTS

Description	Time	Qty

Notes:

Day#:

Time:	Glasses of Water:		CALORIES	FAT	CARBS	PROTEIN	CHOLESTEROL	SODIUM	FIBER
BREAKFAST		**QTY**							
		TOTALS							

Time:	Glasses of Water:		CALORIES	FAT	CARBS	PROTEIN	CHOLESTEROL	SODIUM	FIBER
LUNCH		**QTY**							
		TOTALS							

Time:	Glasses of Water:		CALORIES	FAT	CARBS	PROTEIN	CHOLESTEROL	SODIUM	FIBER
DINNER		**QTY**							
		TOTALS							

CALORIES	FAT	CARBS	PROTEIN	CHOLESTEROL	SODIUM	FIBER

Time: _____   Glasses of Water:

SNACKS   QTY

_____   _____
_____   _____
_____   _____
_____   _____

TOTALS

Daily Totals

CALORIES	FAT	CARBS	PROTEIN	CHOLESTEROL	SODIUM	FIBER

Total Glasses of Water:

RATING

☺
😐
☹

Weight: _____ lbs

EXERCISE/DAILY ACTIVITIES

Description	Time	Qty

VITAMINS/SUPPLEMENTS

Description	Time	Qty

Notes:

Day #: _____

Time: _____ Glasses of Water: ☐

BREAKFAST	QTY	CALORIES	FAT	CARBS	PROTEIN	CHOLESTEROL	SODIUM	FIBER
_____	___							
_____	___							
_____	___							
_____	___							
_____	___ TOTALS							

Time: _____ Glasses of Water: ☐

LUNCH	QTY	CALORIES	FAT	CARBS	PROTEIN	CHOLESTEROL	SODIUM	FIBER
_____	___							
_____	___							
_____	___							
_____	___							
_____	___ TOTALS							

Time: _____ Glasses of Water: ☐

DINNER	QTY	CALORIES	FAT	CARBS	PROTEIN	CHOLESTEROL	SODIUM	FIBER
_____	___							
_____	___							
_____	___							
_____	___							
_____	___							
_____	___ TOTALS							

Date: _____   Day of Week: _____

CALORIES	FAT	CARBS	PROTEIN	CHOLESTEROL	SODIUM	FIBER

Time: _____   Glasses of Water: ☐

SNACKS   **QTY**

_____   _____

_____   _____

_____   _____

_____   _____

TOTALS

Daily Totals

CALORIES	FAT	CARBS	PROTEIN	CHOLESTEROL	SODIUM	FIBER

Total Glasses of Water: ☐

Weight: _____ lbs

RATING

☺

😐

☹

EXERCISE/DAILY ACTIVITIES

Description	Time	Qty

VITAMINS/SUPPLEMENTS

Description	Time	Qty

Notes: _____

_____

_____

Day#:

Time: _____ Glasses of Water:	CALORIES	FAT	CARBS	PROTEIN	CHOLESTEROL	SODIUM	FIBER
BREAKFAST QTY							
_____ ___							
_____ ___							
_____ ___							
_____ ___							
TOTALS							

Time: _____ Glasses of Water:	CALORIES	FAT	CARBS	PROTEIN	CHOLESTEROL	SODIUM	FIBER
LUNCH QTY							
_____ ___							
_____ ___							
_____ ___							
_____ ___							
TOTALS							

Time: _____ Glasses of Water:	CALORIES	FAT	CARBS	PROTEIN	CHOLESTEROL	SODIUM	FIBER
DINNER QTY							
_____ ___							
_____ ___							
_____ ___							
_____ ___							
TOTALS							

Date: | **Day of Week:**

CALORIES	FAT	CARBS	PROTEIN	CHOLESTEROL	SODIUM	FIBER

Time: _____ Glasses of Water: ☐

SNACKS | QTY

_____ _____
_____ _____
_____ _____
_____ _____

TOTALS _____

Daily Totals

CALORIES	FAT	CARBS	PROTEIN	CHOLESTEROL	SODIUM	FIBER

Total Glasses of Water: ☐

Weight: _____ lbs

RATING

☺
😐
☹

EXERCISE/DAILY ACTIVITIES

Description	Time	Qty

VITAMINS/SUPPLEMENTS

Description	Time	Qty

Notes:

Day #:

Time:_____	Glasses of Water: ☐	CALORIES	FAT	CARBS	PROTEIN	CHOLESTEROL	SODIUM	FIBER
BREAKFAST	**QTY**							
_____	__							
_____	__							
_____	__							
_____	__							
	TOTALS							

Time:_____	Glasses of Water: ☐	CALORIES	FAT	CARBS	PROTEIN	CHOLESTEROL	SODIUM	FIBER
LUNCH	**QTY**							
_____	__							
_____	__							
_____	__							
_____	__							
_____	__							
	TOTALS							

Time:_____	Glasses of Water: ☐	CALORIES	FAT	CARBS	PROTEIN	CHOLESTEROL	SODIUM	FIBER
DINNER	**QTY**							
_____	__							
_____	__							
_____	__							
_____	__							
_____	__							
	TOTALS							

Date: | **Day of Week:**

CALORIES	FAT	CARBS	PROTEIN	CHOLESTEROL	SODIUM	FIBER

Time: _____ | **Glasses of Water:** ☐

SNACKS | QTY

_____ _____
_____ _____
_____ _____
_____ _____

TOTALS

Daily Totals

CALORIES	FAT	CARBS	PROTEIN	CHOLESTEROL	SODIUM	FIBER

Total Glasses of Water: ☐

Weight: _____ lbs

RATING

☺
😐
☹

EXERCISE/DAILY ACTIVITIES

Description	Time	Qty

VITAMINS/SUPPLEMENTS

Description	Time	Qty

Notes:

WEEKLY PROGRESS

Clothing size and change in fit:

_____

_____

MEASUREMENTS:

Chest: _____

Waist: _____

Hips: _____

Thigh: _____

Weight: _____

Nutrition/Diet plan followed:
_____%

Physical activity plan followed:
_____%

Weekly Totals						
CALORIES	FAT	CARBS	PROTEIN	CHOLESTEROL	SODIUM	FIBER

This week's achievements:

_____

_____

_____

Changes and adjustments for next week:

_____

_____

_____

DIET TIPS

✓Forgive yourself. If you slip up, renew your commitment and get back on track. Don't let any slip give you an excuse to quit.

✓Experiment with seasonings to perk up repeat foods or to introduce new tastes to your palate.

✓Always leave something on your plate at the end of a meal. Remember to eat until you are satisfied, then stop.

✓Try on new clothes. Notice how your body is changing and appreciate it.

✓Take a cooking class that specializes in the preparation of the foods on your diet.

Day#:

BREAKFAST

Time:	Glasses of Water:							
BREAKFAST	**QTY**	CALORIES	FAT	CARBS	PROTEIN	CHOLESTEROL	SODIUM	FIBER
	TOTALS							

LUNCH

Time:	Glasses of Water:							
LUNCH	**QTY**	CALORIES	FAT	CARBS	PROTEIN	CHOLESTEROL	SODIUM	FIBER
	TOTALS							

DINNER

Time:	Glasses of Water:							
DINNER	**QTY**	CALORIES	FAT	CARBS	PROTEIN	CHOLESTEROL	SODIUM	FIBER
	TOTALS							

Date: **Day of Week:**

CALORIES	FAT	CARBS	PROTEIN	CHOLESTEROL	SODIUM	FIBER

Time: _____   **Glasses of Water:** ☐

SNACKS   QTY

_____ ___

_____ ___

_____ ___

_____ ___

TOTALS

Daily Totals

CALORIES	FAT	CARBS	PROTEIN	CHOLESTEROL	SODIUM	FIBER

Total Glasses of Water: ☐

Weight: _____ lbs

RATING

☺

😐

☹

EXERCISE/DAILY ACTIVITIES

Description	Time	Qty

VITAMINS/SUPPLEMENTS

Description	Time	Qty

Notes:

Day#:

Time: _____	Glasses of Water: ☐	CALORIES	FAT	CARBS	PROTEIN	CHOLESTEROL	SODIUM	FIBER
BREAKFAST	**QTY**							
_____	___							
_____	___							
_____	___							
_____	___							
	TOTALS							

Time: _____	Glasses of Water: ☐	CALORIES	FAT	CARBS	PROTEIN	CHOLESTEROL	SODIUM	FIBER
LUNCH	**QTY**							
_____	___							
_____	___							
_____	___							
_____	___							
	TOTALS							

Time: _____	Glasses of Water: ☐	CALORIES	FAT	CARBS	PROTEIN	CHOLESTEROL	SODIUM	FIBER
DINNER	**QTY**							
_____	___							
_____	___							
_____	___							
_____	___							
	TOTALS							

Date: | Day of Week:

CALORIES	FAT	CARBS	PROTEIN	CHOLESTEROL	SODIUM	FIBER

Time: _____ | Glasses of Water:

SNACKS | QTY

_____ ___
_____ ___
_____ ___
_____ ___

TOTALS

Daily Totals						
CALORIES	FAT	CARBS	PROTEIN	CHOLESTEROL	SODIUM	FIBER

Total Glasses of Water:

Weight:
_____ lbs

RATING

☺

☺

☹

EXERCISE/DAILY ACTIVITIES

Description	Time	Qty

VITAMINS/SUPPLEMENTS

Description	Time	Qty

Notes:

Day #:

Time: ___ Glasses of Water: ☐	CALORIES	FAT	CARBS	PROTEIN	CHOLESTEROL	SODIUM	FIBER
BREAKFAST QTY							
___ ___							
___ ___							
___ ___							
___ ___							
TOTALS							

Time: ___ Glasses of Water: ☐	CALORIES	FAT	CARBS	PROTEIN	CHOLESTEROL	SODIUM	FIBER
LUNCH QTY							
___ ___							
___ ___							
___ ___							
___ ___							
___ ___							
TOTALS							

Time: ___ Glasses of Water: ☐	CALORIES	FAT	CARBS	PROTEIN	CHOLESTEROL	SODIUM	FIBER
DINNER QTY							
___ ___							
___ ___							
___ ___							
___ ___							
___ ___							
TOTALS							

Date: _____   Day of Week: _____

CALORIES	FAT	CARBS	PROTEIN	CHOLESTEROL	SODIUM	FIBER

Time: _____   Glasses of Water: ☐

SNACKS   QTY

_____ ___

_____ ___

_____ ___

_____ ___

TOTALS

Daily Totals

CALORIES	FAT	CARBS	PROTEIN	CHOLESTEROL	SODIUM	FIBER

Total Glasses of Water: ☐

Weight: _____ lbs

RATING

☺

☺/☹ (neutral)

☹

EXERCISE/DAILY ACTIVITIES

Description	Time	Qty

VITAMINS/SUPPLEMENTS

Description	Time	Qty

Notes:

Day #:

Time: _____	Glasses of Water: ☐	CALORIES	FAT	CARBS	PROTEIN	CHOLESTEROL	SODIUM	FIBER
BREAKFAST	**QTY**							
_____	___							
_____	___							
_____	___							
_____	___							
	TOTALS							

Time: _____	Glasses of Water: ☐	CALORIES	FAT	CARBS	PROTEIN	CHOLESTEROL	SODIUM	FIBER
LUNCH	**QTY**							
_____	___							
_____	___							
_____	___							
_____	___							
_____	___							
	TOTALS							

Time: _____	Glasses of Water: ☐	CALORIES	FAT	CARBS	PROTEIN	CHOLESTEROL	SODIUM	FIBER
DINNER	**QTY**							
_____	___							
_____	___							
_____	___							
_____	___							
_____	___							
	TOTALS							

Date:							Day of Week:

CALORIES	FAT	CARBS	PROTEIN	CHOLESTEROL	SODIUM	FIBER

Time: _____ Glasses of Water: ☐

SNACKS   **QTY**

_____ ___
_____ ___
_____ ___
_____ ___

TOTALS

Daily Totals						
CALORIES	FAT	CARBS	PROTEIN	CHOLESTEROL	SODIUM	FIBER

Total Glasses of Water: ☐

Weight: _____ lbs

RATING

☺
😐
☹

EXERCISE/DAILY ACTIVITIES

Description	Time	Qty

VITAMINS/SUPPLEMENTS

Description	Time	Qty

Notes:

Day #:

Time: _____	Glasses of Water: ☐	CALORIES	FAT	CARBS	PROTEIN	CHOLESTEROL	SODIUM	FIBER
BREAKFAST	**QTY**							
_____	___							
_____	___							
_____	___							
_____	___							
	TOTALS							

Time: _____	Glasses of Water: ☐	CALORIES	FAT	CARBS	PROTEIN	CHOLESTEROL	SODIUM	FIBER
LUNCH	**QTY**							
_____	___							
_____	___							
_____	___							
_____	___							
	TOTALS							

Time: _____	Glasses of Water: ☐	CALORIES	FAT	CARBS	PROTEIN	CHOLESTEROL	SODIUM	FIBER
DINNER	**QTY**							
_____	___							
_____	___							
_____	___							
_____	___							
	TOTALS							

Date:							Day of Week:

CALORIES	FAT	CARBS	PROTEIN	CHOLESTEROL	SODIUM	FIBER

Time:_____ Glasses of Water: ☐

SNACKS　　　　　　　　**QTY**

_____ _____

_____ _____

_____ _____

_____ _____

TOTALS

Daily Totals

CALORIES	FAT	CARBS	PROTEIN	CHOLESTEROL	SODIUM	FIBER

Total Glasses of Water: ☐

Weight: _____ lbs

RATING

☺

😐

☹

EXERCISE/DAILY ACTIVITIES

Description	Time	Qty

VITAMINS/SUPPLEMENTS

Description	Time	Qty

Notes:

Day#:

				CALORIES	FAT	CARBS	PROTEIN	CHOLESTEROL	SODIUM	FIBER

Time:_____ Glasses of Water: ☐

BREAKFAST   **QTY**

BREAKFAST	QTY	CALORIES	FAT	CARBS	PROTEIN	CHOLESTEROL	SODIUM	FIBER
_____	___							
_____	___							
_____	___							
_____	___							
TOTALS								

Time:_____ Glasses of Water: ☐

LUNCH	QTY	CALORIES	FAT	CARBS	PROTEIN	CHOLESTEROL	SODIUM	FIBER
_____	___							
_____	___							
_____	___							
_____	___							
_____	___							
TOTALS								

Time:_____ Glasses of Water: ☐

DINNER	QTY	CALORIES	FAT	CARBS	PROTEIN	CHOLESTEROL	SODIUM	FIBER
_____	___							
_____	___							
_____	___							
_____	___							
_____	___							
TOTALS								

114

Date: **Day of Week:**

CALORIES	FAT	CARBS	PROTEIN	CHOLESTEROL	SODIUM	FIBER

Time: _____   Glasses of Water: ☐

SNACKS   QTY

_____   ____

_____   ____

_____   ____

_____   ____

TOTALS

Daily Totals

CALORIES	FAT	CARBS	PROTEIN	CHOLESTEROL	SODIUM	FIBER

Total Glasses of Water: ☐

Weight: _____ lbs

RATING

☺

😐

☹

EXERCISE/DAILY ACTIVITIES

Description	Time	Qty

VITAMINS/SUPPLEMENTS

Description	Time	Qty

Notes:

Day#:

Time: _____	Glasses of Water: ☐

BREAKFAST QTY

	CALORIES	FAT	CARBS	PROTEIN	CHOLESTEROL	SODIUM	FIBER
_____ ____							
_____ ____							
_____ ____							
_____ ____							
TOTALS							

Time: _____	Glasses of Water: ☐

LUNCH QTY

	CALORIES	FAT	CARBS	PROTEIN	CHOLESTEROL	SODIUM	FIBER
_____ ____							
_____ ____							
_____ ____							
_____ ____							
_____ ____							
TOTALS							

Time: _____	Glasses of Water: ☐

DINNER QTY

	CALORIES	FAT	CARBS	PROTEIN	CHOLESTEROL	SODIUM	FIBER
_____ ____							
_____ ____							
_____ ____							
_____ ____							
_____ ____							
TOTALS							

116

Date:							Day of Week:

CALORIES	FAT	CARBS	PROTEIN	CHOLESTEROL	SODIUM	FIBER

Time: _____   Glasses of Water: ☐

SNACKS   QTY

_____ ____

_____ ____

_____ ____

_____ ____

TOTALS

Daily Totals						
CALORIES	FAT	CARBS	PROTEIN	CHOLESTEROL	SODIUM	FIBER

Total Glasses of Water: ☐

Weight: _____ lbs

RATING

☺

😐

☹

EXERCISE/DAILY ACTIVITIES

Description	Time	Qty

VITAMINS/SUPPLEMENTS

Description	Time	Qty

Notes:

WEEKLY PROGRESS

Clothing size and change in fit:
_____

_____

_____

MEASUREMENTS:

Chest: _____

Waist: _____

Hips: _____

Thigh: _____

Weight: _____

Nutrition/Diet plan followed:
_____%

Physical activity plan followed:
_____%

Weekly Totals						
CALORIES	FAT	CARBS	PROTEIN	CHOLESTEROL	SODIUM	FIBER

This week's achievements:
_____

_____

_____

_____

Changes and adjustments for next week:
_____

_____

_____

_____

DIET TIPS

✓ Get rid of your larger-size clothing after losing weight. Claim your commitment to maintaining your weight.

✓ Set a full place setting for yourself when eating. Choose attractive dinnerware and use flowers, candles, cloth napkins, and other items to make your meal time a positive event.

✓ Have a makeover! Discover a new look for yourself.

✓ Remember to be patient and realistic. You did not gain weight overnight and it takes time, effort and focus to lose weight.

Day#:

	QTY	CALORIES	FAT	CARBS	PROTEIN	CHOLESTEROL	SODIUM	FIBER
BREAKFAST Time:_____ Glasses of Water:								
TOTALS								

	QTY	CALORIES	FAT	CARBS	PROTEIN	CHOLESTEROL	SODIUM	FIBER
LUNCH Time:_____ Glasses of Water:								
TOTALS								

	QTY	CALORIES	FAT	CARBS	PROTEIN	CHOLESTEROL	SODIUM	FIBER
DINNER Time:_____ Glasses of Water:								
TOTALS								

Date: _____

Day of Week: _____

CALORIES	FAT	CARBS	PROTEIN	CHOLESTEROL	SODIUM	FIBER

Time: _____ **Glasses of Water:** ⬜

SNACKS	QTY
_____	___
_____	___
_____	___
_____	___
TOTALS	

Daily Totals

CALORIES	FAT	CARBS	PROTEIN	CHOLESTEROL	SODIUM	FIBER

Total Glasses of Water: ⬜

Weight: _____ lbs

RATING

☺

😐

☹

EXERCISE/DAILY ACTIVITIES

Description	Time	Qty
_____	____	___
_____	____	___
_____	____	___
_____	____	___
_____	____	___

VITAMINS/SUPPLEMENTS

Description	Time	Qty
_____	____	___
_____	____	___
_____	____	___
_____	____	___
_____	____	___

Notes:

Day#:

BREAKFAST

Time:_____ Glasses of Water: ▢

QTY

	CALORIES	FAT	CARBS	PROTEIN	CHOLESTEROL	SODIUM	FIBER
_____							
_____							
_____							
_____							
TOTALS							

LUNCH

Time:_____ Glasses of Water: ▢

QTY

	CALORIES	FAT	CARBS	PROTEIN	CHOLESTEROL	SODIUM	FIBER
_____							
_____							
_____							
_____							
TOTALS							

DINNER

Time:_____ Glasses of Water: ▢

QTY

	CALORIES	FAT	CARBS	PROTEIN	CHOLESTEROL	SODIUM	FIBER
_____							
_____							
_____							
_____							
_____							
TOTALS							

Date: _____   Day of Week: _____

CALORIES	FAT	CARBS	PROTEIN	CHOLESTEROL	SODIUM	FIBER

Time: _____   Glasses of Water: ⬜

SNACKS   QTY

_____   _____
_____   _____
_____   _____
_____   _____

TOTALS

Daily Totals

CALORIES	FAT	CARBS	PROTEIN	CHOLESTEROL	SODIUM	FIBER

Total Glasses of Water: ⬜

Weight: _____ lbs

RATING

☺
😐
☹

EXERCISE/DAILY ACTIVITIES

Description	Time	Qty

VITAMINS/SUPPLEMENTS

Description	Time	Qty

Notes:

Day #:

Time: _____	Glasses of Water: ⬜	QTY	CALORIES	FAT	CARBS	PROTEIN	CHOLESTEROL	SODIUM	FIBER
BREAKFAST		QTY							
_____		___							
_____		___							
_____		___							
_____		___							
		TOTALS							

Time: _____	Glasses of Water: ⬜	QTY	CALORIES	FAT	CARBS	PROTEIN	CHOLESTEROL	SODIUM	FIBER
LUNCH		QTY							
_____		___							
_____		___							
_____		___							
_____		___							
_____		___							
		TOTALS							

Time: _____	Glasses of Water: ⬜	QTY	CALORIES	FAT	CARBS	PROTEIN	CHOLESTEROL	SODIUM	FIBER
DINNER		QTY							
_____		___							
_____		___							
_____		___							
_____		___							
_____		___							
		TOTALS							

CALORIES	FAT	CARBS	PROTEIN	CHOLESTEROL	SODIUM	FIBER

Date:

Day of Week:

Time: _____

Glasses of Water: ☐

SNACKS   QTY

_____ ___

_____ ___

_____ ___

_____ ___

TOTALS

Daily Totals

CALORIES	FAT	CARBS	PROTEIN	CHOLESTEROL	SODIUM	FIBER

Total Glasses of Water: ☐

Weight: _____ lbs

RATING

☺

😐

☹

EXERCISE/DAILY ACTIVITIES

Description	Time	Qty

VITAMINS/SUPPLEMENTS

Description	Time	Qty

Notes:

Day #: _____

BREAKFAST

Time: _____ Glasses of Water: ⬜

BREAKFAST	QTY	CALORIES	FAT	CARBS	PROTEIN	CHOLESTEROL	SODIUM	FIBER
_____	___							
_____	___							
_____	___							
_____	___							
TOTALS								

LUNCH

Time: _____ Glasses of Water: ⬜

LUNCH	QTY	CALORIES	FAT	CARBS	PROTEIN	CHOLESTEROL	SODIUM	FIBER
_____	___							
_____	___							
_____	___							
_____	___							
_____	___							
TOTALS								

DINNER

Time: _____ Glasses of Water: ⬜

DINNER	QTY	CALORIES	FAT	CARBS	PROTEIN	CHOLESTEROL	SODIUM	FIBER
_____	___							
_____	___							
_____	___							
_____	___							
_____	___							
TOTALS								

Date: _____   Day of Week: _____

CALORIES	FAT	CARBS	PROTEIN	CHOLESTEROL	SODIUM	FIBER

Time: _____   Glasses of Water: ☐

SNACKS   **QTY**

_____ _____
_____ _____
_____ _____
_____ _____

TOTALS

Daily Totals

CALORIES	FAT	CARBS	PROTEIN	CHOLESTEROL	SODIUM	FIBER

Total Glasses of Water: ☐

Weight: _____ lbs

RATING

☺
😐
☹

EXERCISE/DAILY ACTIVITIES

Description	Time	Qty

VITAMINS/SUPPLEMENTS

Description	Time	Qty

Notes:

Day#:

Time: _____	Glasses of Water: ☐	CALORIES	FAT	CARBS	PROTEIN	CHOLESTEROL	SODIUM	FIBER
BREAKFAST	**QTY**							
_____	___							
_____	___							
_____	___							
_____	___							
	TOTALS							

Time: _____	Glasses of Water: ☐	CALORIES	FAT	CARBS	PROTEIN	CHOLESTEROL	SODIUM	FIBER
LUNCH	**QTY**							
_____	___							
_____	___							
_____	___							
_____	___							
	TOTALS							

Time: _____	Glasses of Water: ☐	CALORIES	FAT	CARBS	PROTEIN	CHOLESTEROL	SODIUM	FIBER
DINNER	**QTY**							
_____	___							
_____	___							
_____	___							
_____	___							
	TOTALS							

Date:

CALORIES	FAT	CARBS	PROTEIN	CHOLESTEROL	SODIUM	FIBER

Time: _____   Glasses of Water: ☐

SNACKS   QTY

_____ ____
_____ ____
_____ ____
_____ ____

TOTALS

Daily Totals

CALORIES	FAT	CARBS	PROTEIN	CHOLESTEROL	SODIUM	FIBER

Total Glasses of Water: ☐

Weight: _____ lbs

RATING

☺

😐

☹

EXERCISE/DAILY ACTIVITIES

Description	Time	Qty

VITAMINS/SUPPLEMENTS

Description	Time	Qty

Notes:

Day#:

BREAKFAST

Time: _____ Glasses of Water: ☐

	CALORIES	FAT	CARBS	PROTEIN	CHOLESTEROL	SODIUM	FIBER
TOTALS							

LUNCH

Time: _____ Glasses of Water: ☐

	CALORIES	FAT	CARBS	PROTEIN	CHOLESTEROL	SODIUM	FIBER
TOTALS							

DINNER

Time: _____ Glasses of Water: ☐

	CALORIES	FAT	CARBS	PROTEIN	CHOLESTEROL	SODIUM	FIBER
TOTALS							

Date: _____ Day of Week: _____

CALORIES	FAT	CARBS	PROTEIN	CHOLESTEROL	SODIUM	FIBER

Time: _____ Glasses of Water: ☐

SNACKS   QTY

_____ _____

_____ _____

_____ _____

_____ _____

TOTALS

Daily Totals

CALORIES	FAT	CARBS	PROTEIN	CHOLESTEROL	SODIUM	FIBER

Total Glasses of Water: ☐

Weight: _____ lbs

RATING

☺

☺

☹

EXERCISE/DAILY ACTIVITIES

Description	Time	Qty

VITAMINS/SUPPLEMENTS

Description	Time	Qty

Notes:

Day#:

Time:_____	Glasses of Water: ☐						
BREAKFAST	**QTY**	CALORIES	FAT	CARBS	PROTEIN	CHOLESTEROL	SODIUM	FIBER
_____	____							
_____	____							
_____	____							
_____	____							
	TOTALS							

Time:_____	Glasses of Water: ☐						
LUNCH	**QTY**	CALORIES	FAT	CARBS	PROTEIN	CHOLESTEROL	SODIUM	FIBER
_____	____							
_____	____							
_____	____							
_____	____							
	TOTALS							

Time:_____	Glasses of Water: ☐						
DINNER	**QTY**	CALORIES	FAT	CARBS	PROTEIN	CHOLESTEROL	SODIUM	FIBER
_____	____							
_____	____							
_____	____							
_____	____							
	TOTALS							

CALORIES	FAT	CARBS	PROTEIN	CHOLESTEROL	SODIUM	FIBER

Time: _____ Glasses of Water: ☐

SNACKS   QTY

_____ ____
_____ ____
_____ ____
_____ ____

TOTALS

Daily Totals

CALORIES	FAT	CARBS	PROTEIN	CHOLESTEROL	SODIUM	FIBER

Total Glasses of Water: ☐

Weight: _____ lbs

RATING

☺
😐
☹

EXERCISE/DAILY ACTIVITIES

Description	Time	Qty

VITAMINS/SUPPLEMENTS

Description	Time	Qty

Notes:

Date: _____ Day of Week: _____

133

WEEKLY PROGRESS

Clothing size and change in fit:
_____
_____
_____

MEASUREMENTS:

Chest: _____
Waist: _____
Hips: _____
Thigh: _____

Weight:_____

Nutrition/Diet plan followed:
_____%

Physical activity plan followed:
_____%

Weekly Totals						
CALORIES	FAT	CARBS	PROTEIN	CHOLESTEROL	SODIUM	FIBER

This week's achievements:
_____
_____
_____
_____

Changes and adjustments for next week:
_____
_____
_____
_____

Nutritive Values of Common Foods and Food Labeling

The success of your diet may be largely dependent on the information you have available. Since the food labeling law became effective in 1994, you can now check the nutritive values of foods found in the supermarket. What follows here are some hints on how to read these:

The expanded nutrition label, called Nutrition Facts, is found on most food packages today. At the top of the label you will find the serving size. Recent efforts have been made by manufacturers to reflect the actual amounts people eat. This number is provided in both household and metric measurements. This is, of course, extemely relevant information because you must make the choice to use the same serving size or compute the difference relevant to the serving size you are using.

The entry for servings per container allows you a better understanding of the serving size based on the entire package. Keep in mind that all of the nutritive value counts are given per serving. The next line reports the calories and gives a second calorie count for the calories from fat.

The list of nutrients that follows on the label represents those thought to be most useful to today's consumer. Total fat, cholesterol, sodium, total carbohydrate and dietary fiber are reported both as the nutritive value count and a percentage. This percentage reflects the Daily Value (DV) and is based on numbers set by the government which reflect the current nutrition recommendations for a 2,000 calorie or a 2,500 calorie diet. You will find the standard used listed in the bottom portion of the label.

Fruits, vegetables, deli and bakery foods with on-site preparation are not required to provide nutrition labels. Also, some foods contain little or no relevant nutrient amounts, therefore no label is required. These products include some spices, coffees and teas. Small packages of food are not required to provide a nutrition label, but must provide a telephone number where consumers can get the information.

Nutrition claims have become very popular in the high-stakes promotion of food items.

Regulations also cover health claims allowed on food packaging. Seven types of health claims are currently allowed, due largely to research linking nutrient and disease prevention:

- Osteoporosis may be prevented by consuming enough calcium
- Limiting sodium intake may help prevent hypertension
- Limiting fat intake may reduce your risk for cancer
- Eating fiber-containing grain products, fruits and vegetables may help prevent cancer
- Eating fruits, vegetables and grain products that contain fiber may help prevent heart disease
- Limiting saturated fat and cholesterol may help reduce the risk of coronary heart disease
- Eating fruits and vegetables may help prevent cancer

FDA requirements for nutrition claims:

Fat Free: Less than 1/2 gram fat
Low fat: 3 grams or less fat (milk can have 5 grams)
Reduced fat: 25% less fat than previous standard for the product
Lite or light: 50% or less fat than previous standard for the product
Sodium free/Salt free: Less than 5 milligrams sodium
Low Sodium: 140 milligrams or less sodium
Very Low Sodium: 35 milligrams or less sodium
High Fiber: 5 grams or more fiber
Cholesterol free: Less than 2 milligrams cholesterol and 2 grams or less saturated fat
Low cholesterol: 20 milligrams or less cholesterol and 2 grams or less saturated fat
Calorie Free: Less than 5 calories
Low calorie: 40 calories or less

The following section provides the nutritive value counts for over 2,000 food items, including many name brands. This reference has been provided to help you easily access the information you need to follow your diet. Now you need only one source to document the progress of your diet.

FOOD	AMOUNT	CAL	FAT	CARB	PROT	CHOL	SOD	FIBER
A								
Acorn squash								
-baked, cubed	1/2 c.	57	.1	14.9	1.1	0	4	2.9
Alfalfa sprouts	1/2 c.	5	.1	.5	.7	0	1	.4
Allspice	1 tsp	5	.2	1.4	.1	0	1	.4
Almond								
-shelled	1/4 c.	210	19	7	7	0	0	2
-slivered	2 oz	170	15	5	6	0	0	2
-roasted	1/3 c.	200	18	6	7	0	200	4
Almond paste								
-*Solo*	2 tbsp	180	11	19	4	0	0	1
Amaranth flour								
-*Arrowhead Mills*	1/4 c.	110	1.5	19	4	0	0	2
Anchovy, canned								
-*Rienzi*								
in soya oil	6 fillets	25	1.5	0	3	15	700	0
Anise seed	1 tsp	7	.3	1.1	.4	0	tr	.3
Antelope	3 oz	127	2	0	na	81	46	0
Apple								
-raw, w/peel	3" diam	96	1	24	.3	0	2	3.7
-dried	2 oz	150	0	42	1	0	40	na
Apple butter								
-*Medford Farms*	1 tbsp	20	0	5	0	0	0	0
Apple cider								
-*Tree Top Frozen*	6 fl oz	90	0	22	0	0	10	na
-*Welch's Sparkling*	6 fl oz	100	0	24	0	0	5	na
Apple juice								
-*Minute Maid*	6 fl oz	80	0	21	0	0	30	na
-*Mott's*	6 fl oz	80	0	20	0	0	10	na
-*Ocean Spray*	6 fl oz	90	0	23	0	0	15	na
-*Red Cheek*	6 fl oz	80	0	20	0	0	10	na
-*Tropicana*	6 fl oz	80	0	20	0	0	15	na

FOOD	AMOUNT	CAL	FAT	CARB	PROT	CHOL	SOD	FIBER
Applesauce								
-Mott's								
sweetened	1/2 c.	100	0	25	0	0	0	1
unsweetened	1/2 c.	50	0	14	0	0	0	1
Apricot								
-fresh	3 med.	55	.2	13.7	1.1	0	1	2.5
-canned								
Del Monte Lite	1/2 c.	60	0	16	0	0	10	1
Apricot, dried								
-Sun Maid	1/4 c.	110	0	25	1	0	0	2
Apricot nectar								
-Libby's	6 fl oz	110	0	26	0	0	0	na
Arrowroot flour	1 c.	457	.1	112.8	.4	0	2	4.4
Artichoke, globe								
-fresh, cooked	1 med.	60	.2	11.9	3.4	0	36	6.5
Artichoke, heart								
-fresh, cooked	1/2 c.	42	.1	9.4	2.9	0	8	4.5
-canned								
Progresso marinated								
w/liquid	1/2 c.	190	15	16	1	0	460	2
Rienzi	1/2 c.	30	0	5	2	0	520	2
-frozen								
Birds Eye	1/2 c.	40	0	8	3	0	45	6
Arugula	1/2 c.	2	.1	.4	.3	0	3	na.
Asparagus	4 spears	12	.1	2.2	1.3	0	1	1.2
Asparagus, canned								
-Del Monte	1/2 c.	20	0	3	2	0	420	1
Avocado								
-California	1 med.	306	30	12	3.6	0	21	4.7
B								
Bacon, Canadian								
-Jones Dairy Farm								
Lean Choice	3 slices	70	3	0	11	30	460	0

FOOD	AMOUNT	CAL	FAT	CARB	PROT	CHOL	SOD	FIBER
-Oscar Mayer	2 slices	50	2	0	9	25	600	0
Bacon, cooked								
-Boar's Head	2 slices	60	5	0	4	10	190	0
-Jones Dairy Farm	2 slices	90	8	0	4	15	350	0
-Oscar Mayer	2 slices	60	5	0	4	10	290	0
"Bacon," vegetarian								
-Morningstar Farms								
Breakfast Strips	3 strips	80	6	4	3	0	350	na
-Worthington								
Stripples	4 strips	120	9	6	4	0	460	na
Bacon bits, imitation								
-Bac*Os	2 tsp	25	1	2	2	0	90	na
-McCormick Bac'N								
Pieces	1 tbsp	26	.5	2	2	na	205	na
Bacon horseradish								
dip								
-Breakstone's	2 tbsp	70	6	2	1	15	279	na
-Kraft	2 tbsp	60	5	2	1	0	200	na
Bagel								
-Thomas'								
Cinnamon Raisin	1 piece	160	1	34	6	0	260	1
Egg	1 piece	160	1	33	7	15	280	1
Onion	1 piece	150	1	33	6	0	280	1
Plain	1 piece	150	1	33	6	0	280	1
Bagel, frozen								
-Lender's								
Blueberry	1 piece	190	2	38	7	0	320	2
Cinnamon raisin	1 piece	190	2	39	6	0	310	2
Egg	1 piece	160	1.5	30	6	0	320	1
Oat	1 piece	170	2	36	7	0	300	4
Onion	1 piece	150	1	30	6	0	300	2
Plain	1 piece	160	1	30	6	0	320	2
Poppy	1 piece	150	1	30	6	0	290	2
Pumpernickle	1 piece	140	1	31	5	0	330	2
Rye	1 piece	140	1	30	5	0	320	2
Sesame	1 piece	150	1	29	6	0	280	2
Soft	1 piece	200	3	38	7	10	340	2

FOOD	AMOUNT	CAL	FAT	CARB	PROT	CHOL	SOD	FIBER
Baked beans								
-Campbell's								
Barbecue	4 oz	130	2	22	5	na	430	6
Brown Sugar								
and Bacon	4 oz	150	3	25	5	na	430	6
Home Style	4 oz	130	2	24	6	na	430	13
Pork and Tomato	4 oz	120	2	21	5	na	370	5
Vegetarian	4 oz	110	1	20	6	0	400	5
Baking mix								
-Bisquick	1/2 c.	240	8	37	4	0	700	na
-Bisquick Reduced								
Fat	1/2 c.	210	4	39	5	0	660	na
Baking powder								
-Davis	1/4 tsp	0	0	0	0	0	95	0
Baking soda								
-Arm & Hammer	1/4 tsp	0	0	0	0	0	119	0
Bamboo shoots,								
canned								
-La Choy	1/4 c.	6	1	1	1	0	2	1
Banana	1 med.	101	.2	26.4	1.3	0	1	2.7
Banana, red	1 med.	118	.3	30.7	1.6	0	1	2.5
Barbecue sauce								
-Heinz Old Fashioned	2 tbsp	40	0	10	0	0	440	0
-KC Masterpiece								
Original	2 tbsp	60	0	13	0	0	210	na
-Kraft Original	2 tbsp	40	0	9	0	0	420	0
-Texas Best								
Original	2 tbsp	40	2.5	4	0	0	430	0
Barley, pearled								
-Arrowhead Mills	1/4 c.	170	.5	37	5	0	0	6
Barley flour								
-Arrowhead Mills	1/4 c.	93	.5	19	3	0	0	3
Basil								
-fresh	1 oz	8	.2	1.2	.7	0	0	na
-dried	1 tsp	4	.1	.9	.2	0	tr.	.2

FOOD	AMOUNT	CAL	FAT	CARB	PROT	CHOL	SOD	FIBER
Bass								
-freshwater	4 oz	129	4.2	0	21.4	77	79	0
-striped	4 oz	110	2.7	0	20.1	91	78	0
Bay leaf, dried	1 leaf	1	0	.1	0	0	1	.1
Beans, dried & canned								
-black beans								
dry								
Goya	1/4 c.	70	0	23	9	0	20	15
canned								
Progresso	4 oz	90	1	19	9	0	350	6.5
-chickpeas								
dry								
Arrowhead Mills	1/4 c.	170	2	29	10	0	10	6
canned								
Goya	1/2 c.	100	2	20	6	0	360	7
-lentils, dry								
Arrowhead Mills								
green	1/4 c.	150	0	27	11	0	15	7
red	1/4 c.	150	0	27	11	0	15	7
-mung beans, dry	1/4 c.	160	.5	28	11	0	0	9
-navy beans								
dry								
Goya	1/4 c.	80	0	23	8	0	15	12
canned	1/2 c.	148	.6	26.8	9.9	0	587	6.7
-pink beans								
dry								
Goya	1/4 c.	70	0	23	8	0	15	15
canned								
Goya	1/2 c.	80	.5	16	5	0	380	7
-pinto beans								
dry								
Arrowhead Mills	1/4 c.	150	.5	27	10	0	0	8
canned								
Goya	1/2 c.	80	1	18	6	0	360	8
-red beans								
canned								
Goya	1/2 c.	90	1	19	7	0	350	8
dried								
Goya	1/4 c.	70	0	22	9	0	20	14
-white beans								
dried								
Goya	1/4 c.	70	0	22	8	0	15	14

FOOD	AMOUNT	CAL	FAT	CARB	PROT	CHOL	SOD	FIBER
canned								
Goya	1/2 c.	100	2	20	6	0	360	6
Beans, fresh								
-cranberry bean,								
boiled	1/2 c.	120	.4	21.5	8.2	0	1	3
-green bean								
fresh	1 c.	43	.2	10	2.4	0	6	3.8
canned								
Green Giant	1/2 c.	20	0	4	1	0	400	1
frozen								
Green Giant	3/4 c.	25	0	5	1	0	0	2
-lima beans								
fresh	1/2 c.	88	.7	15.7	5.3	0	6	3.8
canned								
Del Monte	1/2 c.	80	0	15	4	0	360	4
frozen								
Green Giant	1/2 c.	80	0	15	4	0	130	4
-winged bean								
raw, sliced	1/2 c.	11	.2	1	1.5	0	1	.6
dry	1/2 c.	372	14.9	38	27	0	35	14.1
-yard-long bean								
fresh, sliced	1/2 c.	22	.2	3.8	1.3	0	2	na
Bean dip								
-Hain								
Hot	2 tbsp	40	1	5	2	0	120	na
Mexican	2 tbsp	35	1	5	2	0	120	na
Onion	2 tbsp	35	1	5	2	0	115	na
Beef, choice								
-trimmed brisket								
braised	4 oz	274	14.5	0	33.7	105	79	0
-chuck, arm pot roast								
braised	4 oz	255	10.5	0	37.4	115	75	0
-chuck, blade roast								
braised	4 oz	298	16.3	0	35.2	120	81	0
-flank steak								
broiled	4 oz	256	14.2	0	30	77	92	0
-ground, raw								
extra lean	4 oz	265	19.3	0	21.1	78	75	0
lean	4 oz	298	23.4	0	20	85	78	0
regular	4 oz	351	30	0	18.8	96	77	0
-porterhouse steak								
broiled	4 oz	274	12.2	0	31.9	91	75	0

FOOD	AMOUNT	CAL	FAT	CARB	PROT	CHOL	SOD	FIBER
-rib, whole								
roasted	4 oz	276	15.9	0	30.9	91	82	0
-round, bottom								
braised	4 oz	249	10.7	0	35.8	109	58	0
-round, eye of								
roasted	4 oz	198	6.5	0	32.9	78	70	0
-round, full cut								
broiled	4 oz	217	8.3	0	33.1	88	73	0
-round, top								
broiled	4 oz	214	6.7	0	35.9	95	69	0
-shank								
braised	4 oz	228	7.2	0	38.2	88	73	0
-short ribs								
braised	4 oz	335	20.6	0	34.9	105	66	0
-sirloin, top								
broiled	4 oz	229	9.1	0	34.4	101	75	0
-T-bone steak								
broiled	4 oz	243	11.8	0	31.9	91	75	0
-tenderloin								
broiled	4 oz	252	12.7	0	32	95	71	0
-top loin								
broiled	4 oz	243	11.5	0	32.5	86	77	0
Beef, corned	4 oz	285	21.5	0	20.6	111	1286	0
Beef, corned, hash								
-Dinty Moore	7.5 oz	350	9	22	19	65	850	na
-Libby's	7.5 oz	400	27	20	18	na	1260	na
Beef dishes, frozen								
-Lean Cuisine								
Mesquite, w/rice	1 pkg	280	7	38	16	35	470	6
Oriental	1 pkg	250	8	43	12	15	480	4
Oven Roasted	1 pkg	260	8	28	18	50	590	4
Peppercorn Sirloin	1 pkg	210	7	24	13	25	480	4
Pot Roast, w/Potatoes	1 pkg	210	6	25	13	30	570	6
Salisbury Steak	1 pkg	270	8	27	23	60	590	4
Swedish Meatballs								
w/Pasta	1 pkg	280	7	33	20	50	590	3
-Weight Watchers								
Grilled Salisbury Steak	1 pkg	250	9	24	19	40	590	3
Pepper Steak	1 pkg	240	4.5	33	18	35	690	4
Beef gravy								
-Franco-American	2 oz	35	1	3	2	na	350	na

FOOD	AMOUNT	CAL	FAT	CARB	PROT	CHOL	SOD	FIBER
-Pepperidge Farm	2 oz	25	1	3	2	ma	350	na
Beef jerky								
-Slim Jim								
Big Jerk	1 piece	20	1	1	3	5	170	0
Giant Jerk	1 piece	50	2	2	7	15	420	0
Super Jerk	1 piece	30	1	1	4	10	250	0
Beer								
-regular	12 fl oz	146	0	13.2	.9	0	19	.7
-light	12 fl oz	100	0	.7	4.8	0	10	0
Beet								
-fresh	1/2 c.	29	.1	6.5	1.1	0	40.5	1.9
-canned, w/liquid	1/2 c.	42	.1	9.7	1.1	0	290.5	1.4
Beet green								
-cooked	1 c.	26	.3	4.8	2.5	0	110	na
Biscuit, refrigerated								
-Hungry Jack								
Butter Tastin'	1 piece	90	4	11	2	0	280	na
Buttermilk Flaky	1 piece	90	4	12	2	0	300	na
Buttermilk Fluffy	1 piece	90	4	12	2	0	280	na
Flaky	1 piece	50	1	9	2	0	180	na
Honey Tastin'	1 piece	90	4	13	2	0	290	na
-Pillsbury								
Butter	1 piece	50	1	10	1	0	180	na
Buttermilk	1 piece	50	1	10	1	0	180	na
Country	1 piece	50	1	10	1	0	180	na
Good'N Buttery	1 piece	90	5	11	1	0	270	na
Hearty Grains								
Multi-grain	1 piece	80	2	15	1	0	230	na
Black beans								
-dry								
Goya	1/4 c.	70	0	23	9	0	20	15
-canned								
Progresso	4 oz	90	1	19	9	0	350	6.5
Blackberry								
-fresh	1/2 c.	42	.65	9.3	.85	0	tr.	3.
-canned in syrup								
S & W	1/2 c.	160	0	38	1	0	10	5

FOOD	AMOUNT	CAL	FAT	CARB	PROT	CHOL	SOD	FIBER
Black-eyed peas								
-canned								
Goya	1/2 c.	90	0	19	7	0	380	5
Blintz, frozen								
-Empire Kosher								
Apple	2 pieces	220	5.5	36	6	5	260	5
Bluebery	2 pieces	190	4	36	4	10	260	2
Cheese	2 pieces	200	6	29	11	20	310	3
Cherry	2 pieces	200	4	38	5	10	280	3
Potato	2 pieces	190	6	32	6	10	530	0
Blueberry								
-fresh	1/2 c.	45	.35	11.1	.5	0	1	2
-frozen								
Cascadian Farms	1 c.	90	.5	22	1	0	10	2
-canned								
S&W	1/3 c.	70	0	16	0	0	0	6
Bluefish	4 oz	141	4.8	0	22.7	67	68	0
Bok-choy								
-fresh, shredded	1/2 c.	5	.1	.8	.5	0	23	.4
Bouillon, dry								
-Herb-Ox								
Beef	1 cube	10	0	1	0	0	700	0
Chicken	1 cube	10	0	1	0	0	1040	0
Vegetable	1 cube	10	0	0	0	0	860	0
-Knorr								
Beef	1/2 cube	20	1.5	1	1	na	1290	0
Chicken	1/2 cube	20	1.5	1	1	na	1200	0
Fish	1/2 cube	10	1	0	1	na	960	0
Vegetable	1/2 cube	15	1	1	1	na	910	0
Bratwurst								
-Hillshire Farm								
Fresh	2 oz	190	17	1	7	na	490	0
Fully Cooked	2 oz	170	16	1	7	na	380	0
Smoked	2 oz	190	17	1	8	na	158	0
Brazil nuts	1 oz	185	19	3.1	4.1	0	tr.	1.6

FOOD	AMOUNT	CAL	FAT	CARB	PROT	CHOL	SOD	FIBER
Bread								
-Arnold								
12 Grain Natural	1 slice	60	0	10	2	0	100	1
Bran'nola Country								
Oat	1 slice	90	3	16	2	0	130	3
Bran'nola Dark								
Wheat	1 slice	90	3	15	2	0	150	3
Bran'nola Nutty								
Grain	1 slice	90	2	14	2	0	120	3
Bran'nola Orginal	1 slice	90	2	16	2	0	150	3
Cinnamon Raisin	1 slice	70	1	13	2	0	85	1
French Stick								
Francisco	1 slice	70	2	12	2	0	110	1
Italian Bakery								
Light	1 slice	40	tr	7	2	0	90	2
Italian Francisco	1 slice	70	1	12	2	0	110	na
Oatmeal Bakery	1 slice	60	1	12	2	0	95	2
Oatmeal Bakery								
Light	1 slice	40	tr	8	2	0	100	2
Pita Wheat	1/2 pct.	71	0	16	3	0	na	na
Pita White	1/2 pct.	71	0	16	3	0	na	na
Rye Bakery Soft	1 slice	70	1	14	2	0	170	1
Rye Bakery Soft								
Light	1 slice	40	tr	7	2	0	70	2
Sourdough Francisco	1 slice	90	1	19	2	0	250	1
Wheat Natural	1 slice	80	1	15	2	0	180	2
White Brick Oven	1 slice	60	1	11	2	0	130	1
White Country	1 slice	100	2	18	2	0	200	1
White Extra Fiber								
Brick Oven	1 slice	50	tr	10	2	0	90	2
White Light Brick								
Oven	1 slice	40	tr	10	2	0	95	2
Whole Wheat 100%								
Light Brick Oven	1 slice	40	tr	6	2	0	85	3
-Pepperidge Farm								
Cinnamon	1 slice	90	3	15	2	0	110	2
Cracked Wheat	1 slice	70	1	13	2	0	140	1
Date Walnut	1 slice	90	3	14	2	0	110	2
Honey Bran	1 slice	90	1	18	2	0	160	1
Italian Sliced	1 slice	70	1	12	2	0	125	na
Oatmeal	1 slice	70	1	12	2	0	160	1
Oatmeal Light	1 slice	45	0	9	2	0	95	1
Pumpernickle	1 slice	80	1	15	3	0	230	2
Rye Dijon	1 slice	50	1	9	2	0	180	1
Rye Soft	1 slice	70	1	12	2	0	120	na

FOOD	AMOUNT	CAL	FAT	CARB	PROT	CHOL	SOD	FIBER
Wheat	1 slice	90	2	18	2	0	190	2
Wheat Light	1 slice	45	0	9	2	0	130	2
White Sandwich	2 slices	130	2	24	2	0	260	0
White Toasting	1 slice	90	1	17	2	0	200	1
Whole Wheat Thin Slice	1 slice	60	1	12	2	0	110	2
-Weight Watchers								
Italian	1 slice	38	tr	7	2	0	99	2
Multi-Grain	1 slice	41	1	7	2	0	98	2
Oat	1 slice	42	1	7	2	0	102	2
Raisin	1 slice	55	tr	11	2	0	95	1
Rye	1 slice	38	tr	7	2	0	100	2
Wheat	1 slice	40	tr	7	2	0	99	2
White	1 slice	40	tr	7	2	0	96	2
-Wonder								
White	2 slices	110	1.5	20	3	0	230	1
White, Lite	2 slices	80	1	18	5	0	230	5
Bread crumbs, plain								
Arnold	1 tbsp	50	tr.	8	2	0	80	tr.
4C	1 tbsp	50	1	10	2	0	110	tr.
Bread sticks								
-Stella D'Oro								
garlic	1 piece	35	1	6	1	0	55	na
onion	1 piece	40	1	6	1	0	38	na
plain	1 piece	40	1	7	1	0	55	na
sesame	1 piece	50	2	6	1	0	45	na
Broccoli								
-fresh	1/2 lb	72.5	.7	13.4	8.2	0	34	na
-frozen								
Green Giant	1/2 c.	20	0	4	2	0	115	2
Brownie, ready-to-eat								
-Drake's								
Fudge	1 piece	380	15	60	4	10	102	na
Old Fashioned	1 piece	160	3	20	2	10	100	na
-Hostess Brownie								
Bites	5 pieces	260	14	32	4	50	125	na
-Little Debbie								
Fudge	1 piece	270	13	3	38	11	95	na
Brussels spouts								
-fresh	1/2 c.	19	.1	3.9	1.5	0	11	1.8

FOOD	AMOUNT	CAL	FAT	CARB	PROT	CHOL	SOD	FIBER
-fresh, USDA	1/2 lb	102	.8	18.8	11.1	0	32	NA
Buckwheat flour	1/4 c.	100	1	21	4	0	0	3
Buckwheat groats	1/4 c.	140	1	30	5	0	0	3
Bulgurwheat, dry	1/4 c.	150	.5	33	5	0	0	4
Bun, sweet								
-Entenmann's Fat Free								
Apple	1 bun	150	0	33	3	0	140	1
Cheese and								
Blueberry	1 bun	140	0	31	4	0	150	1
Cheese and								
Pineapple	1 bun	140	0	30	4	0	135	1
Cheese and								
Raspberry	1 bun	160	0	36	4	0	135	0
Cinnamon raisin	1 bun	160	0	36	3	0	125	1
Burrito, frozen								
-Hormel								
Beef	4 oz	300	13	37	9	35	620	na
Cheese	4 oz	250	5	43	9	39	670	na
Chili	4 oz	280	10	40	9	35	620	na
-Old El Paso								
Bean and Cheese	1 piece	330	11	44	14	na	680	na
Beef and Bean								
hot	1 piece	310	11	41	12	na	710	na
med.	1 piece	330	13	41	13	na	630	na
mild	1 piece	320	11	42	13	na	500	na
Butter								
-unsalted	1 tbsp	102	11.5	0	.1	31	1	0
-salted	1 tbsp	102	11.5	0	.1	31	115	0
-whipped, unsalted	1 tbsp	67	7.6	tr.	.1	20	1	0
-whipped, salted	1 tbsp	67	7.6	tr.	.1	20	78	0
Butterfish	4 oz	166	9.1	0	19.6	74	100	0
Butternut squash								
-baked, cubed	1/2 c.	41	.9	10.7	.9	0	4	2.9
Butterscotch chips								
-Nestle Toll House	1 tbsp	80	4	9	0	na	15	0

FOOD	AMOUNT	CAL	FAT	CARB	PROT	CHOL	SOD	FIBER
Butterscotch topping *-Kraft*	1 tbsp	60	1	13	0	0	70	0

C

FOOD	AMOUNT	CAL	FAT	CARB	PROT	CHOL	SOD	FIBER
Cabbage -raw, shredded	1/2 c.	8.5	.4	1.9	.5	0	7	.8
Cabbage, red -raw, shredded	1/2 c.	11	.1	2.4	.5	0	9	.7
Cabbage, savoy -raw, shredded	1/2 c.	8.5	.1	1.6	.85	0	7.5	1.1
Cake *-Entenmann's Fat Free*								
Apple-Spice Crumb	1/8 cake	130	0	30	2	0	140	2
Apricot Danish Twist	1/8 cake	150	0	34	3	0	110	1
Carrot	1/8 cake	170	0	40	3	0	230	1
Chocolate Crunch	1/8 cake	130	0	32	2	0	170	2
Coffee Cinnamon Apple	1/9 cake	130	0	29	2	0	110	2
Golden Crumb	1/8 cake	140	0	35	2	0	150	2
Golden Loaf	1/8 cake	120	0	28	2	0	160	1
Marble Loaf	1/8 cake	130	0	29	2	0	190	1
Raisin Loaf	1/8 cake	140	0	33	2	0	150	1
Cake, frozen *-Sara Lee*								
Cheesecake	1/8 cake	250	16	23	4	20	120	na
Chocolate Mousse	1/8 cake	260	17	23	3	20	100	na
Coconut Layer	1/8 cake	270	14	33	2	20	110	na
Pound	1/15 cake	130	7	14	2	na	85	na
Candy *-3 Musketeers*	2.13 oz	260	8	46	2	5	110	1
-Baby Ruth	2.1 oz	280	12	38	4	0	135	2
-Bit-O-Honey	1.7 oz	200	3.5	41	1	0	105	0
-Butterfinger	2.1 oz	280	11	41	4	0	120	1
-Hershey's milk chocolate	1.5 oz	200	12	21	3	10	30	1
milk chocolate w/ almonds	1.3 oz	210	13	19	4	5	30	1
Kisses	8 pieces	210	12	23	3	10	35	1
Kisses w/almonds	8 pieces	210	13	19	4	5	25	1

FOOD	AMOUNT	CAL	FAT	CARB	PROT	CHOL	SOD	FIBER
-Kit Kat	1.5 oz	220	12	26	3	5	35	1
-M & M's								
almond	1.5 oz	220	12	24	4	5	20	2
peanut	1.5 oz	220	11	25	4	5	20	2
plain	1.5 oz	200	9	30	2	5	30	1
-Milk Duds	1.85 oz	230	8	38	1	0	115	0
-Milky Way	2.15 oz	280	11	43	2	5	90	1
-Raisinets	1.58 oz	200	8	31	2	5	15	2
-Reese's Peanut								
Butter Cup	1.5 oz	250	14	25	5	5	140	1
-Skittles	1.5 oz	170	2	38	0	0	5	0
-Snickers	2.07 oz	280	14	36	4	10	150	1
-Starburst	8 pieces	160	3	33	0	0	20	0
-Twix	1 oz	140	7	19	1	0	60	0
-Twizzler								
strawberry	4 pieces	140	.5	33	1	0	105	0
-York Peppermint								
Pattie	1.5 oz	170	4	33	1	0	15	0
Cantaloupe								
-fresh, cubed	1 c.	48	.2	12	1.1	0	19	NA
Caper								
-Goya								
Spanish	1 tbsp	5	0	1	0	0	380	0
Caramel topping								
-Kraft	1 tbsp	60	0	13	1	0	45	0
Caraway seed	1 tsp	7	.3	1.1	.4	0	tr	.8
Cardamom								
-ground	1 tsp	6	.1	1.3	.2	0	1	.2
-seed	1 tsp	6	.1	1.3	.2	0	tr	.2
Cardoon								
-fresh, shredded	1/2 c.	18	.1	4.4	.6	0	151	1.4
Carissa	1 med.	14	.3	3.2	.1	0	1	.2
Carob drink mix								
-powder	3 tsp	45	tr	11.2	.2	0	12	2
Carob flour	1 c.	395	.7	91.6	4.8	0	36	41

FOOD	AMOUNT	CAL	FAT	CARB	PROT	CHOL	SOD	FIBER
Carp	4 oz	144	6.4	0	20.2	75	58	0
Carrot								
-fresh	1 med.	30	.1	7	.8	0	25	2.2
-fresh, shredded	1/2 c.	23	.1	5.3	.6	0	19	1.7
-frozen, baby								
Masters Choice	1/2 c.	30	0	7	0	0	30	2
-canned, sliced								
Green Giant	1/2 c.	30	0	6	1	0	380	2
Casaba melon								
-fresh, cubed	1 c.	46	tr	11.1	2	0	20	na
Cashew								
-*Planters*	1 oz	170	14	8	5	0	120	1
Cashew butter								
-*Maranatha*	2 tbsp	210	16	8	8	0	9	6
Catfish								
-farmed	4 oz	153	8.6	0	17.7	15	60	0
-wild	4 oz	108	3.2	0	18.6	66	49	0
Cauliflower, florettes								
-fresh, chopped	1 c.	31	.2	5.2	3.1	0	15	2.6
-frozen								
Green Giant	1/2 c.	12	0	3	1	0	25	2
Cavatelli, frozen								
-*Celentano*	3.2 oz	400	1.5	79	16	15	15	9
Caviar								
-black	1 tbsp	40	2.9	.6	3.9	94	240	0
-carp roe	1 tbsp	20	.5	0	3	50	700	0
-lumpfish	1 tbsp	15	1	0	1	50	380	0
-red	1 tbsp	40	2.9	.6	3.9	94	240	0
-salmon	1 tbsp	35	1.5	0	3	55	310	0
-whitefish	1 tbsp	25	1.5	1	1	45	300	0
Celeriac								
-fresh, chopped	1/2 c.	31	.2	7.2	1.2	0	78	1.4
Celery								
-fresh, diced	1/2 c.	10	.1	2.4	.5	0	52	1
Celery salt	1 tsp	6	.4	.6	.3	0	1584	.2

FOOD	AMOUNT	CAL	FAT	CARB	PROT	CHOL	SOD	FIBER
Cereal, hot								
-H-O								
Farina Instant	1 pkg	110	0	22	3	0	235	3
Oatmeal Instant	1 pkg	110	2	18	4	0	230	3
Oat'n Fiber	1 pkg	110	2	18	5	0	140	3
Oat'n Fiber Apple								
& Bran	1 pkg	130	2	26	3	0	140	3
-Quaker								
Oatmeal Instant								
Original	1 pkg	130	3	22	4	0	95	3
Cinnamon Spice	1 pkg	170	2	36	4	0	290	3
Honey Nut	1 pkg	130	3	25	4	0	210	2
Maple Brown								
Sugar	1 pkg	160	2	33	4	0	240	3
Peaches & Cream	1 pkg	130	2	27	4	0	150	2
Raisin Spice	1 pkg	160	2	32	4	0	250	3
Oats, Old Fashioned	1/2 c.	150	3	27	5	0	0	4
Cereal, ready-to-eat								
-General Mills								
Basic 4	3/4 c.	13-	2	28	3	0	290	2
Cheerios	1 c.	110	2	22	3	0	280	3
Cheerios Honey Nut	3/4 c.	110	1	23	3	0	250	2
Fiber One	1/2 c.	60	1	23	3	0	140	13
Kix	1 1/3 c.	120	.5	26	2	0	270	1
Oatmeal Crisp	1/2 c.	110	2	22	2	0	180	1
Total	1 1/3 c.	110	0	26	2	0	280	3
Total Corn Flakes	1 c.	110	tr	24	2	0	200	na
Wheaties	1 c.	110	1	24	3	0	220	3
-Kellogg's								
All Bran	1/2 c.	80	1	22	4	0	280	10
Apple Jacks	1 c.	110	0	26	2	0	135	1
Corn Flakes	1 c.	100	0	24	2	0	300	1
Corn Pops	1 c.	110	0	27	1	0	95	1
Cracklin' Oat Bran	3/4 c.	230	8	40	1	0	180	6
Crispix	1 c.	110	0	26	2	0	230	1
Frosted Flakes	3/4 c.	120	0	28	1	0	200	0
Frosted Mini-Wheats	190	1	45	5	0	0	6	
Nutri-Grain								
Almond Raisin	1 1/4 oz	200	2	44	4	0	330	4
Raisin Bran	1 c.	200	1.5	47	1	0	390	8
Rice Krispies	1 1/4 oz	110	0	26	2	0	320	1
Special K	1 c.	110	0	24	2	0	300	1
-Quaker Oats								
Cap'n Crunch	3/4 c.	110	1.5	23	1	0	210	1

FOOD	AMOUNT	CAL	FAT	CARB	PROT	CHOL	SOD	FIBER
Life	3/4 c.	120	1.5	25	3	0	170	2
-Post								
Fruit & Fiber	1/2 c.	210	3	46	4	0	270	6
Grape Nuts	1/2 c.	200	1	47	6	0	350	5
Grape Nuts Flakes	3/4 c.	100	1	24	3	0	140	3
Cereal, granola								
-C.W. Post Hardy	2/3 c.	280	9	45	5	0	150	4
-Heartland	1/2 c.	290	11	41	9	0	160	4
-Kellogg's Lowfat								
original	1/2 c.	210	3	43	5	0	120	3
raisin	2/3 c.	210	3	43	5	0	135	3
Cheese								
-American	1 oz	105	8.5	.5	6.5	25	na	0
-blue	1 oz	104	8.6	.6	6.1	21	na	0
-Brie	1 oz	100	8	.5	6	28	188	0
-Camembert	1 oz	85	7	.5	5	20	na	0
-cheddar	1 oz	113	9.1	.6	7.1	30	198	0
-Colby	1 oz	110	9	.5	7	27	160	0
-cottage cheese								
Breakstone	1 oz	110	5	3	13	25	370	0
Breakstone 2 %	1 oz	100	2	4	14	15	510	0
Friendship	1 oz	120	5	4	14	17	380	0
Friendship 2%	1 oz	100	2	4	14	9	405	0
Sealtest 2 %	1 oz	100	2	4	15	15	350	0
Light n' Lively 1%	1 oz	80	2	4	14	10	370	0
-cream cheese								
Philadelphia Brand								
regular	1 oz	100	10	1	2	30	90	0
soft	1 oz	100	10	2	1	30	100	0
whipped	1 oz	100	10	1	2	30	85	0
-Edam	1 oz	100	8	.5	7	25	270	0
-farmer	1/2 c.	160	12	4	16	40	356	0
-feta	1 oz	80	6	1	4	25	320	0
-fontina	1 oz	110	9	.5	7	33	na	0
-goat								
hard	1 oz	128	10.1	,6	8,7	30	98	0
semi-soft	1 oz	103	8.5	.7	6.1	22	146	0
soft	1 oz	76	6	.3	5.3	13	104	0
-Gorgonzola	1 oz	93	8	1	5	22	234	0
-Gouda	1 oz	100	8	1	7	32	230	0
-Gruyere	1 oz	117	9.2	.1	8.5	31	95	0
-Havarti	1 oz	120	11	.5	5	31	200	0
-jalapeno jack	1 oz	90	8	1	5	20	430	0

FOOD	AMOUNT	CAL	FAT	CARB	PROT	CHOL	SOD	FIBER
-Jarlsburg	1 oz	100	7	1	7	16	130	0
-Limburger	1 oz	98	7.9	.6	6	26	na	0
-mascarpone	1 oz	128	13.1	1.2	1.5	39	17	0
-Monterey Jack	1 oz	110	9	.5	7	25	150	0
-mozzarella								
whole milk	1 oz	90	7	1	6	25	120	0
part skim	1 oz	80	5	1	8	15	150	0
-Muenster	1 oz	100	9	.5	7	27	180	0
-Neufchatel	1 oz	80	7	1	3	25	115	0
-Parmesan	1 oz	120	7.9	.9	10.9	19	450	0
-Port du Salut	1 oz	100	8	.2	6.7	35	151	0
-pot cheese	1 oz	25	.5	1	5	na	1	0
-provolone	1 oz	100	8	1	7	25	260	0
-queso blanco	1 oz	100	9	.3	7	27	180	0
-queso de papa	1 oz	110	9	.4	7	30	180	0
-ricotta								
whole milk	1 oz	50	4	1	3	15	35	0
part skim	1 oz	45	3	1	4	10	35	0
Polly-O Free	1 oz	25	0	1	4	1	35	0
Polly-O Lite	1 oz	35	2	1	4	5	35	0
-Romano	1 oz	110	8	1	9	29	349	0
-Roquefort	1 oz	105	8.7	.6	6.1	26	513	0
-string								
Frigo	1 oz	80	5	1	7	10	190	0
Polly-O Stick	1 oz	90	6	2	7	15	200	0
-Swiss	1 oz	105	7.9	.5	7.8	26	75	0
"Cheese," nondairy								
-*TofuRella*								
all varieties	1 oz	80	5	2	5	0	290	0
-*Tofutti Better Than Cream Cheese*								
all varieties	1 oz	80	8	1	1	0	135	0
-*VeganRella*								
all varieties	1 oz	60	3	7	1	0	130	.5
-*Zero-FatRella*	1 oz	40	0	3	7	0	250	0
Cherry, maraschino	1 cherry	10	0	2	0	0	0	0
Cherry, sweet								
-fresh, whole	1/2 c.	51	.2	12.6	.95	0	1.5	1.5
Chervil, dried	1 tsp	1	.1	.3	.1	0	1	.1

FOOD	AMOUNT	CAL	FAT	CARB	PROT	CHOL	SOD	FIBER
Chestnut								
-Haddon House	4 nuts	50	0	12	1	0	0	2
Chicken								
-breast w/skin	4 oz	190	12	1	21	80	40	0
-breast, skinless	4 oz	130	3	0	25	75	70	0
-breast, boneless								
and skinless	4 oz	130	2.5	0	25	80	35	0
-ground	4 oz	180	12	0	17	145	65	0
-leg, quarters	4 oz	230	17	1	19	115	70	0
-thigh	4 oz	250	20	0	17	100	80	0
-wing	4 oz	250	20	1	18	125	60	0
"Chicken,"								
vegetarian								
-Worthington								
Chik-Nuggets	5 pieces	240	16	13	12	0	710	5
Chik-Stiks	1 piece	110	7	3	9	0	360	2
Crispy Chik	1 patty	170	9	15	8	0	600	4
Sliced	2 slices	80	4.5	1	9	0	370	1
Chicken coating mix								
-Shake'n Bake								
Barbecue	1/4 pkt	90	2	18	1	0	840	na
Hot and spicy	1/4 pkt	80	2	15	2	0	380	na
Original	1/4 pkt	80	2	14	2	0	450	na
Chicken fat								
-Empire Kosher	1 tbsp	120	13	1	0	10	0	0
Chicken gravy								
-Franco-American	1/4 c.	40	3	3	0	1	240	na
-Heinz Homestyle	1/4 c.	25	1	3	1	1	360	.4
Chicken nuggets								
-refrigerated								
Empire Kosher	5 pieces	180	9	12	13	15	370	1
Perdue	5 pieces	200	12	15	9	35	390	2
-frozen								
Banquet	6 pieces	240	15	12	14	35	540	1
Chicken dishes, frozen								
-Lean Cuisine								
Baked Chicken	1 pkg	230	4	31	18	35	520	5
Breast w/wine Sauce	1 pkg	220	6	25	16	35	560	3

FOOD	AMOUNT	CAL	FAT	CARB	PROT	CHOL	SOD	FIBER
Calypso	1 pkg	280	6	42	15	40	590	3
Carbonara	1 pkg	290	8	32	22	40	540	4
Chow Mein	1 pkg	210	5	28	13	35	510	2
Fettuccine	1 pkg	270	6	33	22	45	580	2
Fiesta	1 pkg	260	5	35	19	40	550	3
Glazed w/vegetable rice	1 pkg	240	6	24	22	60	460	2
Grilled w/Salsa	1 pkg	240	6	32	15	40	550	4
Herb Roasted	1 pkg	210	5	27	13	40	540	3
Honey Mustard	1 pkg	270	5	39	16	35	580	3
Honey Roasted	1 pkg	290	6	46	14	25	590	5
Italian w/fettuccine	1 pkg	270	6	31	22	40	560	3
Mandarin	1 pkg	270	6	41	12	30	520	2
Mediterranean	1 pkg	250	4	35	19	30	570	4
Oriental	1 pkg	260	6	30	21	45	530	3
Parmesan	1 pkg	240	7	25	20	50	580	4
Peanut Sauce	1 pkg	280	6	33	23	45	590	3
Piccata	1 pkg	290	6	45	15	30	540	1
Roasted Herb	1 pkg	210	5	25	17	40	430	4
and Vegetables	1 pkg	240	5	30	19	35	520	5
-Weight Watchers								
BBQ Glazed Chicken	1 pkg	230	2.5	33	20	30	440	4
Cordon Blue	1 pkg	230	4.5	31	15	20	650	2
Fettuccine	1 pkg	290	7	39	19	50	590	4
Parmigiana	1 pkg	310	7	39	21	30	500	4
Penne Pollo	1 pkg	290	5	40	22	35	620	3
Roasted Glazed	1 pkg	240	6	29	18	20	550	4

Chickpea flour
-Arrowhead Mills

FOOD	AMOUNT	CAL	FAT	CARB	PROT	CHOL	SOD	FIBER
-Arrowhead Mills	2 oz	200	3	35	12	0	9	7.4

Chickpeas
-dry

FOOD	AMOUNT	CAL	FAT	CARB	PROT	CHOL	SOD	FIBER
Arrowhead Mills	1/4 c.	170	2	29	10	0	10	6
-canned								
Goya	1/2 c.	100	2	20	6	0	360	7

Chili, canned
-Healthy Choice

FOOD	AMOUNT	CAL	FAT	CARB	PROT	CHOL	SOD	FIBER
w/beans and turkey	7 1/2 oz	200	5	20	18	45	560	na
enchilada flavor	1/2 c.	80	0	15	7	0	160	7
-Hormel								
w/beans	7 1/2 oz	300	28	47	20	92	1010	6
w/beans, chunky	7 1/2 oz	290	14	25	15	50	780	na
w/beans, hot	7 1/2 oz	300	15	27	15	55	1030	na

FOOD	AMOUNT	CAL	FAT	CARB	PROT	CHOL	SOD	FIBER
w/out beans	7 1/2 oz	360	27	14	16	60	860	na
w/out beans, hot	7 1/2 oz	360	27	14	16	60	860	na
Chili, canned, vegetarian								
-Hain								
Spicy	7 1/2 oz	160	1	29	7	0	1060	na
Spicy Tempeh	7 1/2 oz	160	4	24	7	0	1350	na
-Healthy Valley Fat Free								
Bean	1/2 c.	80	0	15	7	0	160	7
3 Bean, mild	5 oz	90	<1	12	10	0	180	9
Black Bean, mild	5 oz	140	<1	23	11	0	290	12.2
Black Bean, hot	5 oz	140	<1	23	11	0	290	12.2
Chili powder	1 tsp	8	.4	1.4	.3	0	26	.9
Chimichanga, frozen								
-Old El Paso								
beef	1 piece	410	25	35	10	na	410	na
chicken	1 piece	370	20	34	13	na	480	na
Chips, corn								
*-Chee*tos*	1 oz	150	9	16	2	0	300	1
-Fritos	1 oz	160	10	15	2	0	150	1
-Sunchips								
Cheddar	1 oz	140	7	18	2	0	180	2
French Onion	1 oz	140	7	18	2	0	115	2
Orginal	1 oz	140	7	18	2	0	160	2
Chips, potato								
-Lay's Baked								
BBQ	1 oz	110	1.5	23	2	0	220	2
Plain	1 oz	110	1.5	23	2	0	150	2
Sour Cream & Onion	1 oz	110	1.5	23	2	0	170	1
-Ruffles								
BBQ	1 oz	150	9	15	1	0	120	1
Cheddar								
& Sour Cream	1 oz	160	10	15	1	0	230	1
Plain	1 oz	150	10	14	2	0	125	1
Plain, Reduced Fat	1 oz	140	6.7	18	2	0	130	1
Ranch	1 oz	150	9	15	2	0	280	1
Sour Cream and								
Onion, Reduced Fat	1 oz	130	6	18	3	0	200	1
-Pringles	1 oz	160	11	15	1	0	170	1
-Pringles Right Crisp	1 oz	140	7	19	2	0	135	1

FOOD	AMOUNT	CAL	FAT	CARB	PROT	CHOL	SOD	FIBER
Chips, tortilla								
-Doritos								
Nacho	1 oz	140	7	18	2	0	170	1
Nacho, Reduced Fat	1 oz	130	5	19	3	0	210	1
Pizza	1 oz	140	7	18	2	0	170	1
Ranch	1 oz	140	7	18	2	0	160	1
Ranch, Reduced Fat	1 oz	130	5	19	2	0	200	1
Toasted	1 oz	140	6	19	2	0	65	1
-Tostitos								
Resturant Style	1 oz	130	6	19	2	0	80	1
Resturant Style, Reduced Fat	1 oz	110	1	24	2	0	200	2
Baked	1 oz	110	1	24	2	0	140	2
Baked Cool Ranch	1 oz	130	3	21	2	3	170	1
Baked Unsalted	1 oz	110	1	24	2	0	0	2
Lime and Chili	1 oz	150	6	19	2	0	80	1
Chips, vegetable								
-Eden								
vegetable chips	1 oz	130	4	24	1	0	260	0
-Terra Chips								
Sweet Potato	1 oz	140	7	18	1	0	10	1
Sweet Potato Spiced	1 oz	140	7	16	1	0	105	3
Taro Spiced	1 oz	130	5	20	1	0	170	2
Vegetable	1 oz	140	7	18	1	0	70	3
Chives								
-fresh, chopped	1 tbsp	1	.1	.2	.1	0	tr.	.1
-dried	1 tbsp	1	.1	.1	.1	0	6	.1
Chocolate, baking								
-Hershey's								
Premium Semi-Sweet	1 oz	140	8	16	1	na	0	na
Premium Unsweetened	1 oz	190	16	7	4	0	5	na
-Nestle								
semi-sweet	1 oz	160	9	16	2	na	0	na
unsweetened	1 oz	180	14	9	4	na	0	na
Chocolate chips								
-Hershey's								
milk	1/4 c.	220	12	27	2	10	55	na
semi-sweet	1/4 c.	220	12	27	1	0	0	na
vanilla	1/4 c.	220	13	25	1	na	100	na

FOOD	AMOUNT	CAL	FAT	CARB	PROT	CHOL	SOD	FIBER
-Nestle								
milk	1 oz	150	7	19	1	na	15	na
semi-sweet	1 oz	140	8	14	2	na	0	4
Chocolate flavor drink (also see "Diet Drinks" and "Health Drinks")								
-Nestle Instant Breakfast	10 fl oz	220	2.5	37	12	5	230	1
-Yoohoo	8 fl oz	130	1	29	2	0	180	0
Chocolate syrup								
-Fox's No Cal	2 tbsp	0	0	0	0	0	35	0
-Hershey's	2 tbsp	110	.1	25	1	0	20	na
Chorizo	1.6 oz	160	13	2	11	45	910	0
Cinnamon, ground	1 tsp	6	.1	1.8	.1	0	1	.6
Clam, raw	4 oz	86	.9	2.3	14.3	39	64	0
Clam, canned								
-Progresso	1/2 c.	40	1	1	8	15	500	0
Clam dip								
-Breakstone's	2 tbsp	50	4	2	1	15	220	na
Clam juice	1 tbsp	0	0	0	0	0	70	0
Cloves, ground	1 tsp	7	.4	1.3	.1	0	5	.7
Cocktail sauce								
-Bennett's	1 tbsp	20	1	4	0	0	260	na
-Sauceworks	1 tbsp	14	0	3	0	0	170	na
Cocoa mix								
-Carnation Fat Free	1 pkt	25	0	4	2	0	135	1
-Swiss Miss								
regular	1 pkt	140	3	27	2	0	130	1
diet	1 pkt	20	0	4	2	0	205	1
fat free	1 pkt	50	0	9	3	0	200	1
-Weight Watchers	1 pkt	70	0	10	6	0	160	1

FOOD	AMOUNT	CAL	FAT	CARB	PROT	CHOL	SOD	FIBER
Cocoa powder								
-Hershey's	1 tbsp	20	.5	3	1	0	0	1
Coconut								
-fresh	1 oz	98	10	2.6	.9	0	6.5	2.6
-packaged, sweetened								
Bakers	2 tbsp	70	5	6	1	0	45	1
Coconut cream								
-canned								
Goya	2 tbsp	140	5	22	0	0	15	0
Coconut milk								
-canned								
Goya	1 oz	93	9	2	2	0	9	0
Cod								
-fresh, Atlantic	4 oz	93	.8	0	20.2	49	62	0
-fresh, Pacific	4 oz	93	.7	0	20.3	42	81	0
Coffee								
-brewed	6 fl oz	4	0	.8	.1	0	4	0
-instant	1 tsp	4	tr	.7	.2	0	1	0
Coffee, mix								
-General Foods International								
Belgian Hazelnut	8 fl oz	70	2	12	1	0	65	0
Cafe Amaretto	8 fl oz	60	3	8	1	0	105	0
French Vanilla	8 fl oz	60	2.5	10	1	0	55	0
Kahlua Cafe	8 fl oz	60	2	10	1	0	55	0
Suisse Mocha	8 fl oz	60	2.5	8	1	0	50	0
Viennese Chocolate	8 fl oz	60	2	10	1	0	30	0
"Coffee," substitute								
-Postum	1 tsp	10	0	3	0	0	110	0
Collards								
-boiled	1 c.	63	1.3	9.7	6.8	0	24	na
Cookie								
-Nabisco								
Apple Newton, Fat Free	2 pieces	100	0	23	1	0	60	1

FOOD	AMOUNT	CAL	FAT	CARB	PROT	CHOL	SOD	FIBER
Chips Ahoy	3 pieces	160	8	23	2	0	105	1
Chips Ahoy, Reduced Fat	3 pieces	140	5	22	2	0	150	1
Cranberry Newton, Fat Free	2 pieces	100	0	23	1	0	95	1
Fig Newton	2 pieces	110	2.5	22	1	0	125	0
Fig Newton, Fat Free	2 pieces	100	0	22	1	0	115	2
Ginger Snaps	4 pieces	120	2.5	22	1	0	230	1
Grahams	8 pieces	120	3	22	2	0	180	1
Nilla Wafers	8 pieces	140	5	24	1	5	100	0
Nilla Wafers, Reduced Fat	8 pieces	120	2	24	1	0	105	0
Nutter Butter	2 pieces	130	6	19	2	>5	110	>1
Oatmeal	1 piece	80	3	12	1	0	65	1
Oreo	3 pieces	160	7	23	1	0	220	1
Oreo Reduced Fat	3 pieces	130	3.5	25	2	0	190	1
Raspberry Newton, Fat Free	2 pieces	100	0	23	1	0	115	1
Vanilla Sandwich	3 pieces	170	8	25	2	0	120	0
Snackwell's								
Fat Free Cinnamon Grahams	1 oz	110	0	26	2	0	90	1
Fat Free Devil's Food	1 piece	50	0	13	1	0	25	tr
Fat Free Double Fudge	1 piece	50	0	12	1	0	70	tr
Reduced Fat Chocolate chip	1 oz	130	4	22	1	0	170	1
Reduced Fat Choc. Sandwich	2 pieces	100	2.5	20	1	0	190	1
Reduced Fat Oatmeal Raisin	2 pieces	110	2	20	1	0	135	1
Reduced Fat Vanilla Sandwich	2 pieces	110	2.5	21	1	0	95	1
Coriander								
-fresh	1/4 c.	1	.1	.1	.1	0	1	.1
-dried	1 tsp	2	.1	.3	.1	0	1	.1
-seed	1 tsp	5	.3	1	.2	0	1	.5
Corn	1 ear	70	.8	16.2	2.5	0	1	2.3

FOOD	AMOUNT	CAL	FAT	CARB	PROT	CHOL	SOD	FIBER
Corn, canned								
-Del Monte								
kernel	1/2 c.	60	1	11	2	0	10	3
kernel, cream-style	1/2 c.	90	.5	20	2	0	360	2
-Hadden House								
baby	1/2 c.	30	1.5	3	1	0	30	4
Corn flour	1 oz	104	.73	21.7	2.2	0	1	3.8
Corn, frozen								
-Birds Eye								
ear	1 ear	140	1.5	34	5	0	20	2
kernel	2/3 c.	80	1	19	3	0	10	1
Cornmeal								
-Arrowhead Mills	1/4 c.	120	1	27	3	0	0	3
Cornstarch	1 tbsp	29	tr	7	tr	0	tr	tr.
Corn syrup								
-Karo								
dark	1 tbsp	60	0	15	0	0	40	0
light	1 tbsp	60	0	15	0	0	30	0
Cornish game hen	3.5 oz	250	15	0	27	155	80	0
Cottage cheese								
-Breakstone	1 oz	110	5	3	13	25	370	0
-Breakstone 2%	1 oz	100	2	4	14	15	510	0
-Friendship	1 oz	120	5	4	14	17	380	0
-Friendship 2%	1 oz	100	2	4	14	9	405	0
-Light n' Lively 1%	1 oz	80	2	4	14	10	370	0
-Sealtest 2%	1 oz	100	2	4	15	15	350	0
Couscous								
-dry	1 oz	107	.2	22	3.6	0	3	1.4
Cowpeas								
-cooked	1 c.	190	.8	34.5	12.8	0	20	na
Crab								
-Alaska king	4 oz	95	.7	0	20.8	47	948	0
-blue	4 oz	99	1.2	.1	20.5	89	332	0
-dungeness	4 oz	98	1.1	.8	19.8	67	335	0
-queen	4 oz	102	1.4	0	21	62	611	0

FOOD	AMOUNT	CAL	FAT	CARB	PROT	CHOL	SOD	FIBER
Crab, canned								
-*Brunswich*	1/4 c.	40	1	0	9	50	240	0
"Crab," imitation	3 oz	70	0	13	6	20	480	1
Crabapple								
-fresh, sliced	1/2 c.	42	.2	11	.2	0	1	.3
Cracker								
-*Carr's Table Water*	5 pieces	70	1.5	13	2	0	100	1
-*Cheez-It*	1 oz	160	8	16	4	0	240	1
-*Cheez-It, Reduced Fat*	1 oz	140	4.5	20	4	0	280	1
-*Club*	4 pieces	70	3	9	1	0	160	0
-*Club, Reduced Fat*	5 pieces	70	2	12	1	0	200	0
-*Devonsheer*								
Melba Toast	3 pieces	50	0	11	2	0	85	1
-*Goldfish*								
cheese	1 oz	140	6	19	4	10	200	1
orginal	1 oz	140	6	19	3	0	230	1
-*J.J. Flats Flatbread*	1 piece	50	1	11	2	0	120	1
-*Krispy*								
fat free	1/2 oz	60	0	12	2	0	135	1
orginal	1/2 oz	60	1.5	10	2	0	180	1
-*Nips*	1 oz	150	6	10	3	0	310	1
-*Oat Thins*	1 oz	140	6	20	3	0	190	2
-*Premium Saltine*								
fat free	1/2 oz	60	0	12	1	0	180	0
orginal	1/2 oz	60	1.5	10	1	0	180	1
-*Ritz*	5 pieces	80	4	10	1	0	135	1
-*Snackwell's*								
Cheese	1 oz	130	2	23	4	0	340	1
-*Stoned Wheat Thins*	2 pieces	60	1.5	10	2	0	140	1
-*Triscuit*								
-*Wheat Thins*	1 oz	140	6	19	2	0	1709	2
Multigrain	1 oz	130	4	21	2	0	290	2
Reduced Fat	1 oz	120	4	21	2	0	220	2
-*Wheatables*	1 oz	150	7	18	3	0	320	1
Cranberry								
-fresh, whole	1/2 c.	22	3.5	5.1	.2	0	1	2
Cranberry bean								
-boiled	1/2 c.	120	.4	21.5	8.2	0	1	3

FOOD	AMOUNT	CAL	FAT	CARB	PROT	CHOL	SOD	FIBER
Cranberry juice								
-*Ocean Spray*								
Cocktail	6 fl oz	100	0	25	0	0	15	0
Cranberry sauce								
-canned, jellied								
Ocean Spray	1/4 c.	110	0	27	0	0	35	1
Crayfish								
-farmed	4 oz	82	1.1	0	16.9	122	70	0
-wild	4 oz	87	1.1	0	18.1	130	66	0
Cream								
-half and half	1 tbsp	20	1.8	.7	.5	6	7	0
-light	1 tbsp	32	3.1	.6	.5	10	6	0
-med., 25% fat	1 tbsp	37	3.8	.5	.4	13	6	0
-whipping, light	1 tbsp	45	4.7	.5	.4	17	5	0
-whipping, heavy	1 tbsp	53	5.6	.5	.3	21	5	0
Cream, sour								
-*Breakstone's*	2 tbsp	60	5	1	1	25	15	0
-*Breakstone's Half*								
and Half	2 tbsp	45	3.5	2	1	15	20	0
-*Breakstone's Free*	2 tbsp	35	0	6	2	5	25	0
-*Friendship*	2 tbsp	55	5	1	1	42	15	0
-*Friendship Light*	2 tbsp	35	2	2	1	8	25	0
Cream, sour, nondairy								
-*Sour Supreme*	2 tbsp	50	5	1	1	0	120	0
Cream cheese								
-*Philadelphia Brand*								
regular	1 oz	100	10	1	2	30	90	0
soft	1 oz	100	10	2	1	30	100	0
whipped	1 oz	100	10	1	2	30	85	0
-*Weight Watchers*	2 tbsp	40	2.5	1	3	10	105	0
Cream cheese substitute								
-*Tofutti Better Than*								
Cream Cheese								
all varieties	1 oz	80	8	1	1	0	135	0
Creamer, nondairy								
-*Coffee-mate*, liquid								
Lite	1 tbsp	10	0	1	1	0	10	0

FOOD	AMOUNT	CAL	FAT	CARB	PROT	CHOL	SOD	FIBER
original	1 tbsp	16	1	2	0	0	5	0
-*Coffee-mate*, powder								
Lite	1 tsp	8	1	2	1	0	0	0
original	1 tsp	10	1	1	1	0	5	0
Croaker	4 oz	119	3.6	0	20.2	69	63	0
Croutons								
-*Pepperidge Farms*								
Caesar	1/2 oz	70	3	8	2	0	180	na
Cheese and Garlic	1/2 oz	70	3	9	2	0	180	na
Italian	1/2 oz	70	3	9	2	0	170	na
Ranch	1/2 oz	70	3	9	2	5	130	1
Seasoned	1/2 oz	70	3	9	2	0	180	na
Cucumber	1 med.	39	.3	9	1.7	0	6	2.4
Cumin seed	1 tsp	8	.5	.9	.4	0	4	.2
Currant								
-fresh	1/2 c.	36	.2	8.6	.8	0	1	3
-dried	1/2 c.	204	.2	53.3	2.9	0	6	4.9
Curry powder	1 tsp	6	.3	1.2	.3	0	1	.7
Cuttlefish	4 oz	90	.8	.9	18.4	127	422	0

D

FOOD	AMOUNT	CAL	FAT	CARB	PROT	CHOL	SOD	FIBER
Dandelion greens								
-fresh, chopped	1/4 lb	51	.8	10.4	3	0	22	1
Date, pitted	10 dates	219	.4	58	1.8	0	1	na
Diet bar								
-*Slim Fast*								
Chewy Caramel	1 bar	120	3.5	22	1	5	45	2
Peanut Caramel	1 bar	120	4	22	1	5	35	1
-*Sweet Success*								
Brownie	1 bar	120	4	23	2	5	35	3
Chocolate chip	1 bar	120	4	23	2	5	40	3
Chocolate raspberry	1 bar	120	4	23	2	5	35	3

FOOD	AMOUNT	CAL	FAT	CARB	PROT	CHOL	SOD	FIBER
Diet drink, liquid								
-Carnation Instant Breakfast								
Chocolate	1 can	220	2.5	37	12	10	230	2
Vanilla	1 can	200	3	31	12	10	180	0
-Slim Fast								
Apple/Cranberry/ Raspberry	1 can	220	1.5	46	7	10	240	5
Chocolate/Straw- berry/Vanilla	1 can	220	3	48	10	5	460	0
Orange/Pineapple	1 can	220	1.5	48	7	10	260	5
-Sweet Success								
Cool Chocolate Mint	10 fl oz	200	2.5	36	10	5	200	3
Creamy Milk Dark Chocolate	10 fl oz	200	2.5	36	10	5	330	3
Fudge	10 fl oz	200	2.5	36	10	5	330	3
Strawberry/Banana	10 fl oz	200	.5	39	9	25	130	4
Strawberry Cream	10 fl oz	200	3	37	10	5	230	3
Vanilla Delight	10 fl oz	200	3	37	10	5	220	3
Diet drink, mix								
-Carnation Instant Breakfast								
Chocolate	1 pkt	70	1	12	4	5	95	1
Vanilla	1 pkt	130	0	27	4	5	130	1
-Crystal Light								
all varieties	1/8 can.	5	0	0	0	0	0	0
-Sweet Success								
Almond	1 pkt	90	1.5	19	7	5	210	6
Chocolate Chip	1 pkt	90	2	19	7	5	100	6
Creamy Milk	1 pkt	90	1.5	19	7	5	210	6
Fudge	1 pkt	90	1.5	19	7	5	210	6
Mocha	1 pkt	90	1.5	19	7	5	210	6
Raspberry	1 pkt	90	1.5	19	7	5	230	6
Dill								
-fresh	1 tbsp	1	.1	.1	1	0	1	.3
-seed	1 tsp	6	.3	1.2	.3	0	tr.	.4
Dolphinfish	4 oz	97	.8	0	21	83	99	0
Drum, freshwater	4 oz	135	5.6	0	19.9	73	85	0
Duck								
-farmed	4 oz	228	12.7	0	26.6	101	74	0

FOOD	AMOUNT	CAL	FAT	CARB	PROT	CHOL	SOD	FIBER
-wild	4 oz	139	4.8	0	22.5	na	65	0
E								
Eel	4 oz	209	13.2	0	20.9	143	58	0
Egg, chicken								
-whole	1 lagre	75	5	.6	6.3	213	63	0
-white only	1 large	17	0	.3	3.5	0	48	0
-yolk only	1 large	59	5.2	.1	2.7	213	9	0
-dried	1 oz	174	12.5	.7	13.7	572	155	0
Egg, duck	1 egg	134	10	.5	9.4	619	102	0
Egg, goose	1 egg	266	19.1	1.9	20	1127	na	0
Egg, quail	1 egg	14	1	.1	1.2	76	na	0
Egg, substitute								
-Egg Beaters	1/4 c.	30	0	1	6	0	100	0
-Egg Watchers	1/4 c.	30	0	1	6	0	80	0
-Morningstar Farms								
Scramblers	1/4 c.	35	0	2	6	0	95	0
Egg, turkey	1 egg	135	9.3	1.3	10.5	737	na	0
Egg roll wrapper								
-Nosoya	2	120	0	24	4	5	290	0
Eggnog								
-Borden	1/2 c.	160	9	17	3	80	80	0
-Borden Light	1/2 c.	150	4	23	5	20	65	0
Eggplant								
-raw, cubed	1 c.	11	.1	2.5	.4	0	1	1
Endive, Belgian								
-fresh, chopped	1/2 c.	8	.1	1.8	.4	0	1	1.4
English muffin								
-Thomas'								
Honey Wheat	1 piece	120	1	21	5	0	200	3
Oat Bran	1 piece	120	1	26	4	0	210	3
Onion	1 piece	130	1	27	4	0	190	2

FOOD	AMOUNT	CAL	FAT	CARB	PROT	CHOL	SOD	FIBER
Raisin Cinnamon	1 piece	151	1	31	4	0	183	2
Regular	1 piece	130	1	25	4	0	210	1
Sour Dough	1 piece	130	1	26	4	0	220	2
Escarole								
-fresh, chopped	1/2 c.	5	.1	1	.4	0	3.5	.8

F

FOOD	AMOUNT	CAL	FAT	CARB	PROT	CHOL	SOD	FIBER
Falafel mix								
-Telma	2 tbsp	110	1	19	5	0	450	4
Fennel								
-bulb, raw, sliced	1/2 c.	27	.2	6.3	1.1	0	45	na
-seed	1 tsp	7	.3	1.1	.3	0	2	.3
Fenugreek seed	1 tsp	12	.2	2.2	.9	0	2	.4
Fig								
-fresh	1 med.	40	.2	10.2	.6	0	1	1.7
-canned								
S&W	5 pieces	140	1	32	0	0	5	3
-dried	1/2 c.	250	2	58	3	0	10	17
Sunmaid	1/4 c.	110	0	26	1	0	0	5
Filberts	1 oz	179	17.6	4.7	3.6	0	tr	1.7
Filbert butter								
-Maranatha	2 tbsp	220	22	6	3	0	0	2
Filo pastry								
-frozen								
Apollo	5 g	180	1	35	5	0	300	1
Flax seeds								
-Arrowhead Mills	3 tbsp	140	10	11	5	0	0	6
Flounder	4 oz	104	1.4	0	21.4	54	92	0
Frankfurter								
-Oscar Mayer								
Beef	1 link	140	13	1	5	25	450	0
Cheese	1 link	140	13	1	5	35	520	0
Wieners	1 link	150	13	1	5	30	450	0

FOOD	AMOUNT	CAL	FAT	CARB	PROT	CHOL	SOD	FIBER
-Oscar Mayer Light								
Beef	1 link	110	9	2	6	25	620	0
Wieners	1 link	110	9	1	7	35	590	0
Frankfurter, chicken								
-Empire Kosher	1 link	100	7	1	8	70	465	0
Frankfurter, turkey								
-Butterball	1 link	130	10	22	7	45	600	0
-Butterball Fat free	1 link	40	0	4	5	15	490	0
-Louis Rich								
and Chicken	1.5 oz	80	6	1	6	40	480	0
and Cheese	1 link	90	7	2	5	40	420	0
"Frankfurter," vege.								
-Morningstar								
Farms Deli Links	1 link	120	7	4	10	0	480	na
-Soy Boy								
Leaner Wieners	1 link	55	0	2	12	0	140	.4
Not Dogs	1 link	95	3	19	7	0	200	0
-Worthington								
Leanies	1 link	100	6	2	8	0	440	na
Frog's legs	4 oz	83	.3	0	18.6	na	na	0
Frosting								
-Pillsbury Supreme								
Chocolate	2 tbsp	140	6	21	0	0	75	0
Chocolate, Dark	2 tbsp	130	6	20	0	0	45	0
Chocolate Fudge	2 tbsp	140	6	21	0	0	80	0
Coconut, Almond	2 tbsp	160	9	18	1	0	60	1
Cream Cheese	2 tbsp	150	6	24	0	0	70	0
Lemon Creme	2 tbsp	150	6	24	0	0	75	0
Strawberry	2 tbsp	150	6	24	0	0	75	0
Vanilla	2 tbsp	150	6	23	0	0	70	0
Fructose	**1 tsp**	**16**	0	4	0	0	0	0
Fruit cocktail, canned								
-Del Monte								
in light syrup	1/2 c.	60	0	15	0	0	10	1
in heavy syrup	1/2 c.	100	0	24	0	0	10	1

FOOD	AMOUNT	CAL	FAT	CARB	PROT	CHOL	SOD	FIBER
G								
Garlic	1 clove	4	.1	.9	.2	0	1	.6
Garlic powder	1 tsp	12	0	2	.5	0	3	na
Garlic salt	1 tsp	5	0	1	.1	0	833	na
Gefilte fish *-Rokeach*	4 pieces	110	6	3	12	25	45	1
Gelatin, dessert, mix *-Jell-O Sugar Free*								
Cherry	1/2 c.	9	0	0	2	0	81	na
Pineapple	1/2 c.	8	tr	0	2	0	50	na
Lemon	1/2 c.	8	0	0	2	0	60	na
Lime	1/2 c.	8	0	0	2	0	63	na
Orange	1/2 c.	8	0	0	2	0	53	na
Peach	1/2 c.	8	tr	0	2	0	49	na
Raspberry	1/2 c.	8	tr	0	2	0	57	na
Strawberry	1/2 c.	9	0	0	2	0	64	na
Gelatin, unflavored *-Knox*	1 pkt	25	0	0	6	0	10	0
Ginger, ground	1 tsp	6	.1	1.3	.2	0	1	.2
Ginger, pickled -Japanese	1 oz	10	.1	1.3	.2	0	1	.2
Ginger, root -trimmed, sliced	1/4 c.	17	.2	3.6	.4	0	3	.5
Goat, roasted	4 oz	162	3.4	0	30.7	85	98	0
Goose, roasted	4 oz	270	14.4	0	32.9	109	86	0
Gooseberry -fresh	1/2 c.	29.5	.15	7.3	.6	0	1	na
-canned w/syrup	1/2 c.	93	.3	23.6	.8	0	3	3

FOOD	AMOUNT	CAL	FAT	CARB	PROT	CHOL	SOD	FIBER
Granola and cereal bars								
-Health Valley Cereal Bars								
all varieties	1 bar	110	0	26	2	0	25	3
-Health Valley Granola Bars								
all varieties	1 bar	140	0	35	2	0	5	3
-Health Valley Healthy Tarts								
all varieties	1 tart	150	0	35	3	0	40	3
-Nutri-Grain								
all varieties	1 bar	140	3	27	2	0	60	1
-Snackwells Cereal Bars								
all varieties	1 bar	120	0	29	1	0	< 140	1
-Snackwells Chewy Granola Bar								
all varieties	1 bar	110	3	22	2	0	40	1
Grape	10 med.	18	.3	4.1	.3	0	1	.3
Grape Juice								
-Welch's								
red	8 fl oz	170	0	44	0	0	20	0
white	8 fl oz	160	0	39	0	0	20	0
Grape leaf, jarred								
-Krinos	1 oz	10	.5	0	1	0	450	2
Grapefruit, fresh								
-California								
red or pink	1/2 med.	46	.1	11.9	.6	0	1	1.4
white	1/2 med.	43	.1	10.7	.6	0	tr.	1.3
-Florida								
red or pink	1/2 med.	38	.1	9.7	.7	0	1	1.4
white	1/2 med.	38	.1	9.2	.7	0	tr.	.2
Green bean								
-fresh	1 c.	43	.2	10	2.4	0	6	3.8
-canned								
Green Giant	1/2 c.	20	0	4	1	0	400	1
-frozen								
Green Giant	3/4 c.	25	0	5	1	0	0	2
Grenadine syrup	1 tbsp	32	1	8	1	0	14	0

FOOD	AMOUNT	CAL	FAT	CARB	PROT	CHOL	SOD	FIBER
Grits								
-Quaker Quick Grits	1/4 c.	130	.5	29	3	0	0	2
Grouper	4 oz	104	1.2	0	22	42	60	0
Guava	1/2 c.	42	.5	10.7	.7	0	2	4.9
Guinea hen								
-without skin	4 oz	125	2.8	0	23.4	71	na	0
H								
Haddock	4 oz	99	.8	0	21.5	65	78	0
Halibut	4 oz	124	2.6	0	23.6	37	61	0
Ham, canned								
-Black Label	1 oz	37	1	<2	5	15	303	0
-Hormel								
Curemaster	2 oz	60	2	1	10	26	627	0
-Oscar Mayer	2 oz	60	2	1	10	26	450	0
Ham, cured								
-whole leg, lean w/fat								
unheated	4 oz	279	21	.1	21	64	1456	0
-whole leg, lean only								
unheated	4 oz	167	6.5	.1	25.3	59	1719	0
-boneless, 11% fat								
unheated	4 oz	206	12	3.5	19.9	65	1493	9
-boneless, 5% fat								
unheated	4 oz	149	5.6	1.1	21.9	53	1620	0
Ham, fresh								
-leg, roasted	4 oz	333	23.5	0	28.4	105	67	0
-rump, roasted	4 oz	311	20.2	0	30.2	108	69	0
-shank, roasted	4 oz	344	25.1	0	27.6	104	66	0
Ham and cheese Pocket sandwich								
-Hot Pockets	4.5 oz	350	16	36	16	55	790	na
-Weight Watchers								
Ultimate 200	4 oz	200	6	24	14	5	490	na

FOOD	AMOUNT	CAL	FAT	CARB	PROT	CHOL	SOD	FIBER
"Hamburger," vege-								
tarian, frozen								
-Amy's California	1 patty	100	3	17	4	0	290	3
-Green Giant								
Harvest Burgers								
Italian	1 patty	140	4.5	8	17	0	370	5
Original	1 patty	140	4	8	18	0	270	5
Southwestern	1 patty	140	4	9	16	0	370	5
-Morningstar Farms								
Better'n Burgers	1 patty	70	0	6	11	0	360	3
Garden Grain	1 patty	120	2.5	18	6	5	280	4
Garden Veggie	1 patty	100	2.5	9	10	0	350	4
Grillers	1 patty	140	7	5	14	0	260	3
"Hamburger,"								
vegetarian, mix								
-Fantastic Foods	1/3 c.	170	1.5	34	7	0	580	5
-Nature's Burger								
Original	3 oz	155	3	26	6	0	287	4
BBQ	3 oz	133	1	26	5	0	430	3
Pizza	3 oz	133	1	26	5	1	431	0
Health bar								
-Balance Bar								
all varieties	1 bar	190	6	22	14	5	<240	0
-Cliff Bar								
Chocolate Chip	1 bar	250	3	51	4	0	45	3
Chocolate Chip/								
Peanut Butter	1 bar	250	6	40	12	0	110	5
Chocolate/Espresso	1 bar	250	2	52	4	0	100	2
Dark Chocolate	1 bar	250	2	52	5	0	20	2
-Power Bar								
all varieties	1 bar	230	2.5	45	10	0	<110	3
-Pure Protein								
Chocolate	1 bar	250	4	13	30	5	80	1
Peanut Butter	1 bar	280	7	9	33	5	80	0
-Tiger Sport Bar								
Chocolate Blast	1 bar	230	3	40	11	0	100	na
Coffee Rush	1 bar	230	3	40	11	0	90	na
Vanilla Blast	1 bar	220	2	40	11	0	125	na
Health drink, liquid								
-Boost								
all varieties	1 can	240	4	40	10	5	130	0

FOOD	AMOUNT	CAL	FAT	CARB	PROT	CHOL	SOD	FIBER
-Ensure								
all varieties	1 can	225	6	31	12	5	290	1
-Ensure Plus								
all varieties	1 can	360	13	47	13	5	250	0
-Nutrament								
all varieties	1 can	360	10	52	16	5	250	0
Health drink, mix								
-Twin Lab								
Diet Fuel	1 scoop	120	0	9	20	0	30	0
Egg Fuel	1 scoop	110	0	2	25	0	390	0
Pro-Fuel Chocolate	3 scoops	296	1	34	40	0	50	na
Pro-Fuel Strawberry	3 scoops	296	1	34	40	0	50	na
Vege-Fuel	2 scoops	120	1	0	30	0	na	na
Herring, fresh								
-Atlantic	4 oz	180	10.3	0	20.4	68	102	0
-Pacific	4 oz	224	15.8	0	18.6	87	84	0
Herring, jarred								
-Elf								
cream sauce	3 oz	167	10	7	12	42	798	0
dill sauce	3 oz	152	8	10	10	38	832	0
horseradish sauce	3 oz	218	16	11	8	40	1512	0
Hollandaise sauce mix								
-French's	1/5 pkg	25	1	4	1	20	240	na
-Knorr	1 serving	16	.3	2.6	.5	<1	140	na
Hominy, canned								
-Allens golden	1/2 c.	80	<1	16	2	0	350	na
-Allens white	1/2 c.	70	<1	16	2	0	430	na
Honey	1 tbsp	64	0	17.3	.1	0	1	0
Honeydew, melon								
-fresh, cubed	1/2 c.	56	.5	13.1	1.4	0	20	1
Horseradish, fresh								
-chopped	1/2 c.	19	.1	.8	.9	0	1	.2
Horseradish, prepared								
-Kraft	1 tbsp	10	0	1	0	0	140	na
-Gold's hot	1 tbsp	4	<1	<1	<1	0	60	na
-Gold's red	1 tbsp	4	0	<1	<1	0	75	na

FOOD	AMOUNT	CAL	FAT	CARB	PROT	CHOL	SOD	FIBER
-Gold's white	1 tbsp	4	< 1	< 1	< 1	0	55	na
Hummus mix								
-Casbah	1 oz	120	5	12	5	0	200	na
I								
Ice cream								
-Breyers								
Butter pecan	1/2 c.	180	12	15	3	25	125	na
Cherry Vanilla	1/2 c.	150	7	17	3	20	45	0
Chocolate	1/2 c.	160	8	20	3	20	30	0
Chocolate Mint	1/2 c.	170	10	18	3	25	45	0
Coffee	1/2 c.	150	8	16	3	30	50	0
Strawberry	1/2 c.	130	6	16	2	20	40	0
Vanilla	1/2 c.	150	8	15	3	25	50	0
-Edy's Grand								
Butter Pecan	1/2 c.	160	9	17	3	27	50	na
Chocolate	1/2 c.	160	9	16	2	31	30	0
Chocolate Chip	1/2 c.	160	9	18	3	24	45	0
Coffee	1/2 c.	140	8	15	3	30	41	0
Strawberry	1/2 c.	130	6	16	3	20	35	0
Vanilla	1/2 c.	160	10	14	2	40	30	0
-Weight Watchers								
Chocolate, Triple	1/2 c.	150	3.5	26	4	5	80	1
Cookie Dough	1/2 c.	140	3.5	24	3	5	85	1
Praline	1/2 c.	140	3	25	3	5	105	0
Rocky Road	1/2 c.	140	3	23	4	5	75	1
Vanilla	1/2 c.	120	2.5	20	4	5	65	1
"Ice cream," rice								
-Rice Dream								
all varieties	1/2 c.	170	8	26	1	0	95	1
"Ice cream," substitute								
- Healthy Choice								
Chocolate	1/2 c.	130	2	24	3	5	70	0
Chocolate Chip	1/2 c.	130	2	24	3	5	70	0
Coffee Toffee	1/2 c.	130	2	25	3	5	80	0
Fudge Swirl	1/2 c.	130	2	24	3	5	70	0
Rocky road	1/2 c.	160	2	32	3	5	70	0
Vanilla	1/2 c.	120	2	21	4	5	60	0

FOOD	AMOUNT	CAL	FAT	CARB	PROT	CHOL	SOD	FIBER
"Ice Cream," tofu								
-Tofutti								
Chocolate	1/2 c.	180	11	18	3	0	180	0
Vanilla	1/2 c.	190	11	20	2	0	210	0
Vanilla almond	1/2 c.	210	13	21	3	0	130	0
Vanilla fudge	1/2 c.	190	9	25	2	0	130	0
-Tofutti Fruitti								
all fruit flavors	1/2 c.	100	0	20	2	0	90	0
-Tofutti Low Fat								
Chocolate Fudge	1/2 c.	120	2	25	2	0	98	0
Coffee Marshmallow	1/2 c.	100	1	24	1	0	77	0
Strawberry Banana	1/2 c.	100	1	23	1	0	92	0
Vanilla Fudge	1/2 c.	120	2	24	2	0	90	0
Ice cream bar								
-Dove								
chocolate, dark								
chocolate coated	1 bar	350	22	34	4	41	40	na
chocolate, milk								
chocolate coated	1 bar	340	21	35	4	42	60	na
vanilla, dark								
chocolate coated	1 bar	340	22	33	4	40	45	na
vanilla, milk								
chocolate coated	1 bar	340	21	33	5	40	45	na
-Haagen-Dazs								
chocolate, dark								
chocolate coated	1 bar	380	27	38	5	85	60	na
fudge	1 bar	210	14	19	4	75	50	na
vanilla, dark								
chocolate coated	1 bar	380	27	38	5	90	65	na
vanilla, milk								
chocolate coated	1 bar	330	24	25	5	90	75	na
"Ice cream bar," rice								
-Rice Dream								
Cappuccino	1 bar	130	5	19	1	0	70	1
Carob	1 bar	130	5	20	1	0	70	1
Carob Almond	1 bar	140	6	20	1	0	85	2
Chocolate	1 bar	270	15	32	2	0	95	2
Cookies 'n Dream	1 bar	140	6	21	1	0	70	1
Lemon	1 bar	130	5	19	1	0	70	1
Peanut Butter Fudge	1 bar	130	6	21	2	0	75	1
Strawberry	1 bar	110	5	18	1	0	65	1
Vanilla	1 bar	130	5	19	1	0	70	1
Vanilla Fudge	1 bar	130	5	19	1	0	70	1

FOOD	AMOUNT	CAL	FAT	CARB	PROT	CHOL	SOD	FIBER
Ice milk								
-Light n' Lively								
Carmel Nut	1/2 c.	120	4	18	3	10	85	na
Chocolate Chip	1/2 c.	120	4	18	3	10	35	na
Coffee	1/2 c.	100	3	16	3	10	40	na
Cookies n' Cream	1/2 c.	110	3	20	3	10	35	na
Vanilla	1/2 c.	100	3	16	3	10	45	na
Vanilla Fudge Twirl	1/2 c.	110	3	18	3	10	45	na
J								
Jams and preserves,								
-all varieties								
Knott's Berry Farm	1 tsp	18	0	4	0	0	0	na
Kraft	1 tsp	17	0	4	0	0	0	na
Polaner	2 tsp	35	0	9	0	0	0	na
Smucker's	1 tsp	18	0	4	0	0	0	na
-grape								
Welch's	2 tsp	35	0	9	0	0	5	na
Jelly								
-all flavors								
Knott's Berry Farm	1 tsp	18	0	4	0	0	0	na
Kraft	1 tsp	17	0	4	0	0	0	na
Polander	2 tsp	35	0	9	0	0	0	na
Smucker's	1 tsp	18	0	4	0	0	0	na
Welch's	2 tsp	35	0	9	0	0	5	na
Jerusalem artichoke								
-fresh, sliced	1/2 c.	57	.1	13.1	1.5	0	na	1.2
K								
Kale								
-cooked, chopped	1/2 c.	21.5	.4	3.3	2.5	0	15	1
Kamut								
-Arrowhead Mills	1/4 c.	110	.5	25	4	0	0	4
Ketchup								
-Heinz	1 tbsp	15	0	4	0	0	190	0
-Hunt's	1 tbsp	15	0	4	0	0	200	0
-Muir Glen Organic	1 tbsp	15	0	3	0	0	190	0

FOOD	AMOUNT	CAL	FAT	CARB	PROT	CHOL	SOD	FIBER
Kielbasa								
-*Healthy Choice*	2 oz	70	1.5	6	7	20	480	0
-*Hillshire Farm*	2 oz	190	17	2	7	25	460	0
Kiwifruit	1 med.	46	.3	11.3	.8	0	4	2.6
Knockwurst								
-*Hillshire Farm*	2 oz	180	16	1	7	na	460	0
Kohlrabi								
-fresh, sliced	1/2 c.	20.5	.1	4.6	1.4	0	5.5	2.5
Kumquat	1 med.	12	tr	3.2	.2	0	1	1.3
L								
Lamb, choice								
-foreshank, braised, lean only	4 oz	212	6.8	0	35.2	118	84	0
-ground	4 oz	320	25.5	0	18.8	83	67	0
-leg, roasted, lean only	4 oz	217	8.8	0	32.1	101	77	0
-loin chop, broiled, lean only	4 oz	245	11	0	34	108	95	0
-rib, roasted	4 oz	263	15.1	0	29.7	100	92	0
-shoulder, roasted	4 oz	231	12.2	0	28.3	99	77	0
Lard, pork	1 tbsp	115	12.8	0	0	12	tr.	0
Leek								
-fresh, chopped	1/2 c.	32	.2	7.4	.8	0	10	.9
Lemon	1 med.	20	.2	6	.8	0	1	na
Lemon juice								
-fresh	1 tbsp	4	tr	1.2	.1	0	tr.	.1
-bottled, *ReaLemon*	1 tbsp	0	0	0	0	0	0	0
Lemon peel	1 tbsp	tr	.1	1	.1	0	tr	.6
Lemonade								
-*Minute Maid*	8 fl oz	110	0	31	0	0	25	0
-*Tropicana*	8 fl oz	120	0	29	0	0	20	0

FOOD	AMOUNT	CAL	FAT	CARB	PROT	CHOL	SOD	FIBER
Lentil, dry								
-Arrowhead Mills								
green	1/4 c.	150	0	27	11	0	15	7
red	1/4 c.	150	0	27	11	0	15	7
Lettuce								
-bib or Boston,								
chopped	1 c.	8	.1	1.4	.7	0	5	.8
-cos or romaine,								
chopped	1 c.	10	.2	1.9	.7	0	5	3
-iceberg,								
chopped	1 c.	7	.1	1.6	.5	0	5	.7
Lima beans								
-fresh	1/2 c.	88	.7	15.7	5.3	0	6	3.8
-canned								
Del Monte	1/2 c.	80	0	15	4	0	360	4
-frozen								
Green Giant	1/2 c.	80	0	15	4	0	130	4
Lime	2" diam	19	.1	6.4	.5	0	1	.8
Lime juice								
-fresh	1 tbsp	4	tr	1.4	.1	0	tr.	.1
-bottled, *ReaLime*	1 tbsp	0	0	0	0	0	0	0
-sweetened, *Rose's*	1 tbsp	24	1	6	1	0	3	0
Liquor								
80 proof	1 fl oz	65	0	tr.	0	0	tr.	0
86 proof	1 fl oz	70	0	tr.	0	0	tr.	0
90 proof	1 fl oz	74	0	tr.	0	0	tr.	0
100 proof	1 fl oz	83	0	tr.	0	0	tr.	0
Liver								
-beef, braised	3 oz	137	4	3	22	331	59	0
-chicken, simmered	4 oz	187	5	1	30	716	58	0
-duck, raw	4 oz	39	1.3	1	5.3	146	na	0
-goose, raw	4 oz	38	1.2	1.8	4.6	na	40	0
-pork, braised	4 oz	187	5	4.3	29.5	403	56	0
-turkey, simmered	4 oz	197.2	5.4	3.5	31.6	710	62.2	0
-veal, braised	4 oz	187	7.8	4.8	3.1	24.5	636	0
Lobster, cooked								
-bite size	4 oz	107	1.7	.3	21.1	108	238	0

FOOD	AMOUNT	CAL	FAT	CARB	PROT	CHOL	SOD	FIBER
"Lobster," imitation	2 oz	50	1	5	6	na	320	0
Lobster sauce								
-Progresso	1/2 c.	120	8	11	4	10	430	0
Luncheon meats								
-Boar's Head								
bologna	2 oz	150	13	0	7	35	530	0
brisket	2 oz	80	3	0	12	40	460	0
chicken, roasted	2 oz	50	1	1	11	30	420	0
chicken, smoked	2 oz	60	1	1	11	30	440	0
ham	2 oz	60	1	2	9	25	90	0
ham, Black Forest	2 oz	60	.5	2	10	30	580	0
ham, maple	2 oz	60	1	3	10	20	570	0
ham, pepper	2 oz	70	2	3	9	30	590	0
ham, Virginia	2 oz	60	1	3	9	25	590	0
roast beef	2 oz	90	3	0	14	30	40	0
turkey	2 oz	60	1.5	1	12	35	360	0
turkey, hickory								
smoked	2 oz	70	2	1	12	25	340	0
turkey, maple								
honey	2 oz	70	.5	2	14	30	440	0
turkey, oven								
roasted	2 oz	60	2	0	11	25	340	0
turkey pastrami	2 oz	60	.5	0	14	30	390	0
salami	2 oz	120	9	0	10	25	470	0
salami, Genoa	2 oz	180	14	1	12	55	970	0
-Oscar Mayer								
bologna	1 oz	90	8	0	3	20	270	0
chicken, roasted,								
Fat Free	1.8 oz	45	0	1	9	25	650	0
ham, baked	3 slices	60	1	2	11	30	720	0
ham, boiled	3 slices	60	2.5	0	10	30	820	0
ham, honey	3 slices	70	2.5	2	10	30	760	0
ham, smoked	3 slices	60	2.5	0	10	30	750	0
roast beef, Deli-thin	4 slices	60	1.5	1	11	25	530	0
turkey	1 oz	30	1	1	4	10	330	0
salami	2 slices	120	10	1	6	30	510	0
salami, dry	3 slices	100	9	0	6	25	510	0
salami, Genoa	3 slices	100	9	0	5	25	490	0
spiced loaf	1 oz	70	5	2	4	20	340	0
-Louis Rich								
turkey, BBQ	2 oz	60	1	2	2	25	630	0
turkey, hickory								
smoked	2 oz	60	.5	1	11	25	740	0

FOOD	AMOUNT	CAL	FAT	CARB	PROT	CHOL	SOD	FIBER
turkey, honey roasted	2 oz	60	.5	2	11	25	660	0
turkey, oven roasted	2 oz	50	.5	1	11	25	620	0
turkey ham	2 oz	70	2.5	1	11	40	620	0
turkey pastrami	2 oz	70	2	1	11	40	590	0
turkey salami	2 oz	120	9	1	8	50	500	0
Lychees, shelled	5 fruits	29	.1	7.4	.4	0	1.5	.5

M

FOOD	AMOUNT	CAL	FAT	CARB	PROT	CHOL	SOD	FIBER
Macadamia nut -*Mauna Loa*	1 oz	220	22	3	2	0	60	2
Macadamia nut butter -*Maranatha*	2 tbsp	230	24	5	3	0	0	3
Macaroni, cooked	1 c.	155	.6	32.2	4.8	0	1	na
Macaroni and cheese, frozen								
-*Lean Cuisine*	9 oz	290	9	37	15	30	550	na
-*Stouffer's*	6 oz	250	13	23	11	na	640	na
-*Weight Watchers*	1 pkg	300	7	49	11	10	570	2
Macaroni and cheese, mix								
-*Kraft*	3/4 c.	290	13	34	9	5	530	na
Mace, ground	1 tsp	8	.6	.9	.1	0	1	.3
Mackerel, fresh								
-Atlantic	4 oz	232	15.8	0	21.1	80	102	0
-king	4 oz	119	2.3	0	23	61	179	0
-Pacific and jack	4 oz	179	9	0	22.8	53	98	0
-Spanish	4 oz	158	7.2	0	21.9	86	67	0
Mahi mahi	4 oz	97	.8	0	21	83	99	0
Mango								
-peeled, sliced	1 c.	109	.7	27.7	1.2	0	12	3
Manicotti								
-*Celentano*	7 oz	410	19	31	19	100	630	7

FOOD	AMOUNT	CAL	FAT	CARB	PROT	CHOL	SOD	FIBER
Maple syrup	1 tbsp	50	0	13.2	0	0	1.8	0
Maple syrup, imitation								
-*Aunt Jemima*	1/4 c.	210	0	54	0	0	170	0
-*Log Cabin*	1 oz	103	0	27	0	0	22	0
Margarine								
-*Land OLakes*	1 tbsp	100	11	0	0	0	100	0
-*Mazola*	1 tbsp	100	11	0	0	0	100	0
-*Mazola Light*	1 tbsp	50	6	0	0	0	130	0
-*Parkay*	1 tbsp	100	11	0	0	0	105	0
-*Parkay Squeeze*	1 tbsp	80	9	0	0	0	110	0
-*Weight Watchers*	1 tbsp	60	7	0	0	0	130	0
Marjoram, dried	1 tsp	2	.1	.4	.1	0	tr	.1
Marshmallow								
-*Campfire*	2 lrg	40	0	10	0	0	10	na
-*Kraft Jet-Puffed*	5 lrg	110	0	27	0	0	27	0
-*Kraft Miniature*	1/2 c.	100	0	25	0	0	30	0
-*Fluff*	1 tsp	59	tr	14	0	0	12	na
Matzo								
-*Manischewitz*								
American	1 cracker	115	1.9	22	2.9	0	na	na
Egg	1 cracker	132	2	27	4	25	5	na
Passover	1 cracker	129	.4	27	3.3	0	5	na
Whole Wheat	1 cracker	110	.6	21	4	0	1	.6
Mayonnaise								
-*Hellman's*	1 tbsp	100	11	0	0	5	80	0
-*Hellman's Light*	1 tbsp	50	5	1	0	5	115	0
-*Kraft*	1 tbsp	100	11	0	0	5	75	0
-*Kraft Fatfree*	1 tbsp	32	0	2	0	0	120	0
Mayonnaise, canola								
-*Smartbeat Light*	1 tbsp	40	4	1	0	0	110	0
"Mayonnaise," imitation								
-*Miracle Whip*								
fat free	1 tbsp	15	0	3	0	0	120	0
light	1 tbsp	40	3	3	0	0	120	0
salad dressing	1 tbsp	70	7	2	0	5	85	0
"Mayonnaise," tofu								
-*Nayonaise*	1 tbsp	35	3	1	0	0	105	0

FOOD	AMOUNT	CAL	FAT	CARB	PROT	CHOL	SOD	FIBER
Milk								
-whole, 3.3%	8 oz	150	8	12	8	35	130	0
-2%	8 oz	130	5	12	8	20	130	0
-1%	8 oz	100	2.5	11	8	10	130	0
-skim	8 oz	80	0	12	8	3	130	0
Milk, buttermilk	8 oz	110	4	11	9	20	110	0
Milk, canned								
-condensed, sweet	1 tbsp	61	1.7	10.4	1.5	66	24	0
Carnation	2 tbsp	130	3	22	3	10	45	0
-evaporated								
Carnation	1/2 c.	170	10	12	8	37	135	0
Carnation Lite	1/2 c.	100	1	14	9	5	150	0
Carnation lowfat	1/2 c.	110	3	12	8	10	140	0
Milk, dry								
-Fearn Non-Fat	3 tbsp	90	0	13	9	0	130	0
Milk, goat's	1 c.	163	9.8	11.2	7.8	28	83	0
Milkfish	4 oz	168	7.6	0	23.3	59	na	0
Millet, whole								
-Arrowhead Mills	1/4 c.	150	1.5	34	5	0	0	3
Millet flour								
-Arrowhead Mills	1/4 c.	110	1	26	4	0	0	2
Miso								
-Eden	1 tbsp	35	2	2	3	na	600	na
Molasses								
-Brer Rabbit Dark	1 tbsp	60	0	14	0	0	15	0
-Grandma's gold	1 tbsp	68	1	17	1	0	28	0
Monkfish	4 oz	86	1.7	0	16.4	29	21	0
Monosodium glutamate	1 tsp	0	0	0	0	0	638	0
Mousse, frozen								
-Weight Watchers chocolate	1 serving	190	5	31	6	5	150	3

FOOD	AMOUNT	CAL	FAT	CARB	PROT	CHOL	SOD	FIBER
Muffin								
-Entenmann's Fat Free								
blueberry	1 piece	120	26	2	0	0	220	1
Muffin, frozen								
-Weight Watchers								
banana nut	1 piece	180	4	34	3	15	260	5
blueberry	1 piece	160	0	38	3	0	290	2
chocolate								
chocolate chip	1 piece	190	2	39	2	0	350	4
Mullet, striped	4 oz	133	4.3	0	22	56	74	0
Mung beans, dry	1/4 c.	160	.5	28	11	0	0	9
Mushroom								
-fresh, sliced	1 c.	20	.2	3.1	1.9	0	2	.8
-canned	1/4 c.	12	0	2	1	0	220	1
B in B	1/2 c.	30	0	4	3	0	460	2
Mushroom								
-enoli	1 oz	10	.1	2.2	.4	0	1	na
-oyster	1 oz	7	.1	1.3	.6	0	1	.2
-portobello	1 oz	8	.8	1.2	.1	0	4	1
-shiitake	1oz	48	.3	3.2	2.1	0	na	.7
Mussel, meat only	4 oz	98	2.5	4.2	13.5	32	324	0
Mustard, prepared								
-brown								
Heinz Spicy	1 tsp	14	1	1	1	0	115	0
-Dijon								
Grey Poupon	1 tsp	18	1	0	0	0	450	0
-mild								
Heinz	1 tsp	8	1	1	1	0	175	0
-stone ground								
Hain	1 tsp	14	1	1	1	0	185	na
-yellow								
French's	1 tsp	10	1	1	1	0	180	na
Mustard greens								
-cooked, chopped	1/2 c.	16	.3	2.8	1.5	0	7	.6
Mustard powder	1 tsp	9	.6	.3	.5	0	1	.1

FOOD	AMOUNT	CAL	FAT	CARB	PROT	CHOL	SOD	FIBER
Mustard seed	1 tsp	15	1	1.2	.8	0	tr	.2
Mustard spinach -cooked, chopped	1/2 c.	14.5	.2	2.5	1.5	0	na	.8

N

FOOD	AMOUNT	CAL	FAT	CARB	PROT	CHOL	SOD	FIBER
Navy Bean -dry								
Goya	1/4 c.	80	0	23	8	0	15	12
-canned	1/2 c.	148	.6	26.8	9.9	0	587	6.7
Nectarine	1 med.	88	tr	23.6	.8	0	tr	2.2
New Zealand spinach -cooked, chopped	1/2 c.	11	.2	1.9	1.5	0	37	.2
Noodle, Chinese								
-cellophane, dry	2 oz	199	.1	48.8	.1	0	6	.1
-chow mein	1/2 c.	150	8	16	3	0	230	1
-rice	1/2 c.	130	5	21	2	0	420	1
Noodle, egg, dry	2 oz	220	2.6	40.8	7.3	55	2.8	na
Noodle, Japanese								
-soba, dry	2 oz	192	.4	42.5	8.2	0	451	na
-somen, dry	2 oz	203	.5	42.2	6.5	1	1049	2.4
-udon, dry	2 oz	159	.7	32.3	3.9	0	340	na
Nutmeg, ground	1 tsp	12	.8	1.1	.1	0	tr	.5

O

FOOD	AMOUNT	CAL	FAT	CARB	PROT	CHOL	SOD	FIBER
Oat flour -Arrowhead Mills	1/3 c.	120	2	20	5	0	0	4
Oats, dry -groats								
Arrowhead Mills	1/4 c.	160	3	29	6	0	0	4
-rolled or oatmeal	1 oz	109	1.8	19	4.5	0	1	2.9
-steel cut								
Arrowhead Mills	1/4 c.	170	3	29	6	0	0	0

FOOD	AMOUNT	CAL	FAT	CARB	PROT	CHOL	SOD	FIBER
Ocean perch	4 oz	107	1.9	0	21.1	48	85	0
Octopus	4 oz	93	1.2	2.5	16.9	55	na	0
Oil								
-almond	1 tbsp	120	13.6	0	0	0	0	0
-avocado	1 tbsp	124	14	0	0	0	0	0
-cocoa butter	1 tbsp	120	13.6	0	0	0	0	0
-coconut	1 tbsp	117	13.6	0	0	0	0	0
-cod liver	1 tbsp	123	13.6	0	0	78	na	0
-corn	1 tbsp	120	13.6	0	0	0	0	0
-cottonseed	1 tbsp	120	13.6	0	0	0	0	0
-hazelnut	1 tbsp	120	13.6	0	0	0	0	0
-herring	1 tbsp	123	13.6	0	0	104	na	0
-oat	1 tbsp	120	13.6	0	0	0	0	0
-olive	1 tbsp	120	14	0	0	0	0	0
-palm	1 tbsp	120	13.6	0	0	0	0	0
-palm kernel	1 tbsp	120	13.6	0	0	0	0	0
-peanut	1 tbsp	120	14	0	0	0	0	0
-poppyseed	1 tbsp	120	13.6	0	0	0	0	0
-safflower	1 tbsp	120	14	0	0	0	0	0
-salmon	1 tbsp	123	13.6	0	0	66	na	0
-sardine	1 tbsp	123	13.6	0	0	97	na	0
-sesame	1 tbsp	120	14	0	0	0	0	0
-soybean	1 tbsp	120	14	0	0	0	0	0
-sunflower	1 tbsp	120	14	0	0	0	0	0
-vegetable	1 tbsp	120	14	0	0	0	0	0
-walnut	1 tbsp	120	14	0	0	0	0	0
Oil spray								
-Pam								
Butter Flavor	1 spray	2	tr	0	0	0	0	0
Olive Oil	1 spray	2	tr	0	0	0	0	0
Plain	1 spray	2	tr	0	0	0	0	0
-Weight Watchers								
Butter Flavor	1 spray	2	tr	0	0	0	0	0
Plain	1 spray	2	tr	0	0	0	0	0
Okra								
-fresh, sliced	1 c.	36	.3	7.6	2.4	0	3	2.6
Olive								
-Krinos								
Calamata	1/2 oz	40	4	2	0	0	260	0
green	1/2 oz	15	1	1	0	0	410	0

FOOD	AMOUNT	CAL	FAT	CARB	PROT	CHOL	SOD	FIBER
ripe, oil cured	1/2 oz	70	6	3	0	0	390	0
ripe, salt cured	1/2 oz	30	2.5	1	0	0	310	0
-*Vlasic*								
Spanish	1/2 oz	14	0	1	0	na	300	na
Onion								
-fresh, chopped	1/2 c.	32.5	.1	7.4	1.3	0	2	1.4
Onion, green								
-fresh, chopped	1/2 c.	18	.1	4.1	.8	0	2	na
Onion, jarred								
-cocktail								
Hanover	1/2 c.	23	0	6	1	0	420	1
Onion powder	1 tsp	8	.1	1.7	.2	0	1	.1
Onion salt	1 tsp	1	tr	.4	.1	0	1599	.1
Orange								
-California navel	3" diam	87	.2	21.8	2.2	0	2	3.4
-California Valencia	3" diam	96	.4	15	1.4	0	1	2.9
-Florida	3" diam	89	.4	22.6	1.3	0	2	3.6
Orange, canned								
-*Dole Mandarin*	1/2 c.	80	0	19	0	0	10	0
Orange juice								
-fresh	1 c.	112	.5	25.8	1.7	0	2	na
-chilled								
Minute Maid	6 fl oz	80	0	20	1	0	20	na
Tropicana	6 fl oz	80	1	16	1	0	20	na
-frozen								
Minute Maid	6 fl oz	80	0	20	1	0	0	na
Oregano, dried	1 tsp	6	.1	1	.2	0	1	.2
Oyster, fresh								
-Eastern	4 oz	76	2	3	7.2	na	63	0
Oyster, canned								
-drained	4 oz	74	2	3.8	9.5	62	82	0

FOOD	AMOUNT	CAL	FAT	CARB	PROT	CHOL	SOD	FIBER
P								
Palm hearts, canned								
-*Goya*	1/2 c.	25	.5	4	2	0	450	2
Pancake, frozen								
-*Aunt Jemima*								
Lowfat	3 pieces	130	1.5	33	4	0	580	8
Original	3 pieces	200	3	40	6	15	700	2
-*Hungry Jack*								
Microwave	3 pieces	240	4	47	5	10	550	2
Pancake syrup								
-*Aunt Jemima*								
Lite	1/4 c.	100	0	26	0	0	160	0
Original	1/4 c.	210	0	53	0	0	120	0
Papaya								
-fresh, cubed	1/2 c.	27.5	.1	7	.4	0	2	1.3
Paprika	1 tsp	6	.3	1.2	.3	0	1	.4
Parsley								
-fresh, chopped	1 tbsp	2	tr	.3	.1	0	2	1
-dried	1 tsp	1	.1	.2	.1	0	1	.1
Parsley root	1 oz	3	.2	.7	.8	0	28	.4
Parsnip								
-boiled, diced	1/2 c.	51	.4	11.6	1.1	0	6	3.3
Passion fruit	1 med.	16	.1	3.9	.4	0	2.5	1.9
Pasta, dry								
-*Creamette*								
all varieties	2 oz	210	1	42	7	0	0	2
-*Masters Choice*								
all varieties	2 oz	210	1	41	7	0	0	2
-*Ronzoni*								
all varieties	2 oz	210	1	42	7	0	<7	2
Pasta, refrigerated								
-*Contadina*	3 oz	260	4	45	12	75	35	na

FOOD	AMOUNT	CAL	FAT	CARB	PROT	CHOL	SOD	FIBER
Pasta dishes, frozen								
-Lean Cuisine								
Chicken Marinara	1 pkg	270	6	38	15	20	540	4
Marinara Twist	1 pkg	240	3	42	10	5	440	4
Spaghetti								
w/Meatballs	1 pkg	280	6	40	16	20	570	4
and Tuna Casserole	1 pkg	280	6	39	18	20	590	4
and Turkey Dijon	1 pkg	270	6	37	16	30	570	6
-Weight Watchers								
Bow Ties w/								
Mushroom								
Marsala Sauce	1 pkg	280	9	36	13	10	560	5
Cheese Manicotti	1 pkg	260	7	31	17	30	570	5
Pasta and Spinach								
Romano	1 pkg	240	8	32	11	5	510	4
Penne w/Sundried								
Tomatoes	1 pkg	290	9	41	12	15	560	4ss
Penne w/Tomato								
Basil Sauce	1 pkg	260	9	33	12	10	260	5
Pasta sauce								
-Hunt's Chunky	4 oz	50	1	12	1	0	470	2
-Prego	4 oz	120	4	20	2	na	540	na
-Progresso	4 oz	110	5	13	3	5	660	na
-Ragu Old World	4 oz	100	3	15	2	0	460	na
Pasta sauce, meat								
-Hunt's	4 oz	70	2	12	2	2	570	2
-Prego	4 oz	120	4	20	2	na	580	na
-Progresso	4 oz	110	5	13	4	5	660	na
-Ragu Old World	4 oz	80	5	7	2	2	740	na
Pastrami								
-Hillshire Farm	1 oz	31	.4	1	6	na	290	0
Peach								
-fresh, sliced	1/2 c.	32.5	.1	8.9	.6	0	1	1.7
Peach, canned								
-America's Choice								
in heavy syrup	1/2 c.	100	0	24	1	0	10	1
Peach, frozen								
-Big Valley	2/3 c.	50	0	13	1	0	0	2

FOOD	AMOUNT	CAL	FAT	CARB	PROT	CHOL	SOD	FIBER
Peanut, shelled								
-Planters								
cocktail	1 oz	170	14	6	7	0	115	2
dry-roasted	1 oz	160	13	6	7	0	190	2
Peanut butter								
-Jiff	2 tbsp	190	16	7	8	0	150	2
-Jiff Simply	2 tbsp	190	16	6	8	0	65	2
-Smuckers Natural								
chunky & creamy	2 tbsp	200	16	7	7	0	120	2
Reduced Fat	2 tbsp	200	12	12	9	0	120	2
Peanut butter flavor								
baking chips	1/4 c.	230	13	19	9	5	90	na
Peanut flour								
-defatted	1 c.	223	5.5	18.9	28.7	0	5	2.4
Pear								
-fresh, sliced	1/2 c.	50.5	.35	12.6	.6	0	1	2
Pear, canned								
-Del Monte								
canned, light syrup	1/2 c.	60	0	15	0	0	10	1
canned, heavy syrup	1/2 c.	100	0	24	0	0	10	1
Pear, Asian	1 med.	51	.3	13	.6	0	0	4.4
Peas, green								
-fresh, shelled	1/2 c.	61	.3	10.5	4.5	0	1.5	3.7
Peas, green, canned								
-Del Monte	1/2 c.	60	0	11	3	0	10	4
Peas, green, frozen								
-Green Giant	3/4 c.	70	0	13	4	0	220	4
Peas, snow								
-fresh	1/2 c.	30	.1	5.4	2	0	3	1.9
Pecan, shelled								
-pieces	1/3 c.	200	20	4	3	0	0	2
Pectin, unsweetened								
-dry	1 pkg	163	.1	45.2	.1	0	100	na

FOOD	AMOUNT	CAL	FAT	CARB	PROT	CHOL	SOD	FIBER
Pepper, banana								
-*Vlasic*	1 oz	4	0	1	0	0	480	na
Pepper, cherry								
-*Vlasic*	1 oz	8	0	2	0	0	480	na
Pepper, chili								
-fresh, green or								
red, chopped	1/2 c.	30	.2	7.1	1.5	0	5	1.1
Pepper, ground								
-black	1 tsp	5	.1	1.4	.2	0	1	.6
-cayenne	1 tsp	6	.3	1	.2	0	1	.5
-chili	1 tsp	9	.3	1.4	.3	0	1	.3
-white	1 tsp	7	.1	1.7	.3	0	tr	.1
Pepper, jalapeno								
-*Ortega*	1 oz	10	0	3	0	0	20	na
Pepper, pepperoncini								
-*Progresso*	1/2 c.	20	0	7	0	0	5	1
Pepper, sweet								
-green								
fresh, chopped	1/2 c.	16.5	.1	3.6	.9	0	1	.9
-red								
fresh, chopped	1/2 c.	23.5	.2	5.3	1	0	1	.9
-jarred								
Progresso roasted	1/2 c.	20	0	5	1	0	2	1.7
Pepper sauce, hot								
-*Pickapeppa*	1 tbsp	4	0	4	0	0	95	na
-*Tabasco*	2 fl oz	7	.2	.7	.4	0	404	0
Pepperoni								
-*Oscar Mayer*	1 oz	140	25	13	0	6	550	0
Perch	4 oz	103	1.1	0	22	102	70	0
Persimmon								
-Japanese, fresh	1 med.	129	.7	33.1	1.2	0	na	6
- native, fresh	1 med.	31	.1	8.2	.2	0	tr	.4
Pheasant								
-with skin	4 oz	205	10.5	0	25.7	na	45	0

FOOD	AMOUNT	CAL	FAT	CARB	PROT	CHOL	SOD	FIBER
Pickle								
-bread and butter								
Vlasic	1 oz	25	0	6	0	0	170	na
-dill								
Vlasic	1 oz	4	0	1	0	0	390	na
-hamburger chips								
Vlasic	1 oz	4	0	1	0	0	180	na
-sour	1 oz	3	.1	.6	.1	0	342	.3
-sweet								
Vlasic	1 oz	45	0	10	0	0	170	na
Pie filling, canned								
-*Comstock apple*	1/3 c.	90	0	22	0	0	75	2
-*Comstock*								
blueberry	1/3 c.	100	0	25	0	0	15	1
-*Comstock cherry*	1/3 c.	90	0	23	0	0	25	1
-*Libby's pumpkin*	1 c.	260	.3	64	2	0	440	na
Pierogi, frozen								
-*Golden Potato and*								
Cheese	3 pieces	250	8	38	8	35	260	2
-*Golden Potato and*								
Onion	3 pieces	210	6	36	6	na	220	1
Pigeon peas								
-fresh	1/2 c.	105	1.3	18.4	5.5	0	4	3.2
Pike								
-northern	4 oz	100	.8	0	21.8	44	44	0
-walleye	4 oz	105	1.4	0	21.7	98	58	0
Pimiento, jarred	1 oz	7.5	.3	3.3	.5	0	na	na
Pine nuts								
-pignoli	1 oz	156	13.4	3.3	8.8	0	na	1.3
-pinyon	1 oz	180	17.2	5.8	3.7	0	na	1
Pineapple								
-fresh, diced	1/2 c.	40.5	.2	10.6	.3	0	1	.9
Pineapple, canned								
-*Dole*								
canned, in juice	2 slices	60	0	15	0	0	10	1
canned, in syrup	2 slices	90	0	23	0	0	10	1

FOOD	AMOUNT	CAL	FAT	CARB	PROT	CHOL	SOD	FIBER
Pink bean								
-dry								
Goya	1/4 c.	70	0	23	8	0	15	15
-canned								
Goya	1/2 c.	80	.5	16	5	0	380	7
Pinto bean								
-dry								
Arrowhead Mills	1/4 c.	150	.5	27	10	0	0	8
-canned								
Goya	1/2 c.	80	1	18	6	0	360	8
Pistachio								
-salted	30 nuts	170	15	8	4	0	260	3
Pistachio butter								
-Maranatha	2 tbsp	200	17	9	5	0	0	4
Pizza, French bread, frozen								
-Healthy Choice								
Cheese	5.6 oz	290	4	46	19	15	390	na
Deluxe	6.35 oz	330	7	41	23	35	50	na
Pepperoni	6 oz	310	7	38	20	30	470	na
-Lean Cuisine								
3 Cheese	5.5 oz	330	10	38	23	20	350	na
Cheese	5 1/8 oz	300	9	38	17	310	na	
Deluxe	6 1/8 oz	350	11	40	22	30	580	na
Pepperoni	5.25 oz	340	11	41	19	25	580	na
Pizza, frozen								
-Weight Watchers								
Cheese	6.03 oz	300	7	36	24	10	310	na
Pepperoni	6.03 oz	320	8	36	25	15	550	na
Pizza crust								
-Pillsbury All Ready	1/8 crust	90	1	16	3	0	170	na
Plantain	1 large	313	1.1	82	2.9	0	7	4.1
Plum								
-Damson, fresh, sliced	1/2 c.	56	tr	15.1	.4	0	1.5	1.2
-Japanese or hybrid fresh, sliced	1/2 c.	39.5	.2	10.2	.4	0	1	1.2

FOOD	AMOUNT	CAL	FAT	CARB	PROT	CHOL	SOD	FIBER
Plum, canned								
-S & W	1/2 c.	130	0	33	0	0	15	2
Polenta								
-San Gennaro	100 g	70	0	15	2	0	310	1
Pollock								
-Atlantic	4 oz	104	1.1	0	22.1	80	98	0
-walleye	4 oz	91	.9	0	19.5	81	112	0
Pomegranate	1 med.	97	.5	25.3	.8	0	5	.9
Pompano	4 oz	186	10.7	0	21	57	74	0
Popcorn								
-Orville Redenbacher								
Original	2 tbsp	90	1	22	3	0	0	5
Hot air	2 tbsp	90	1	23	4	0	0	5
Microwave								
Butter	2 tbsp	170	12.5	15	2	0	390	4
Butter light	2 tbsp	120	5.5	19	3	0	350	4.6
Caramel	2 tbsp	180	10	23	1	0	50	2
Cheddar	2 tbsp	140	9	16	2.5	5	285	4
Movie Theater	2 tbsp	180	13	16	2	0	500	4
Movie Theater								
Light	2 tbsp	115	5	19	3	0	320	4.5
Natural	2 tbsp	160	11	17.5	2	0	510	4
Original	2 tbsp	120	6	19	3	0	350	5
Poppyseed	1 tsp	15	1.3	.7	.5	0	1	.8
Pork								
-loin, whole								
roasted, lean only	4 oz	272	15.8	0	30.5	102	78	0
-loin, blades								
roasted, lean only	4 oz	316	21.9	0	28	101	77	0
-loin, center								
roasted, lean only	4 oz	272	14.8	0	32.3	103	78	0
-loin, top								
roasted, lean only	4 oz	278	15.6	0	32	90	52	0
-shoulder, whole								
roasted, lean only	4 oz	277	17	0	28.8	110	86	0
-shoulder, Boston								
roasted, lean only	4 oz	290	19.1	0	27.6	110	83	0

FOOD	AMOUNT	CAL	FAT	CARB	PROT	CHOL	SOD	FIBER
-sirloin								
roasted, lean only	4 oz	268	14.9	0	31.2	102	70	0
-spareribs, braised,								
lean w/fat	6.3 oz	703	53.6	0	51.4	214	165	0
-tenderloin								
roasted, lean only	4 oz	188	5.5	0	32.6	105	76	0
Pork seasoning and coating mix								
-Shake'n Bake								
BBQ	1/8 pkg	35	0	8	0	0	260	na
Hot and Spicy	1/8 pkg	45	1	8	1	0	220	na
Orginal	1/8 pkg	40	1	8	1	0	310	na
Pork skins, fried	1 oz	160	10	2	12	25	850	na
Potato	1 med.	86	.1	19.2	2.4	0	3	1.8
Potato, canned								
-Allens Whole	1/2 c.	50	1	10	1	0	230	1.8
Potato, mashed, mix								
-Hungry Jack	1/3 c.	80	0	18	2	0	45	1
-Pillsbury	2 tbsp	90	0	20	2	0	25	2
Potato pancake, frozen								
-Golden	1 piece	80	3	11	2	5	210	1
Pretzel								
-hard, plain	1 oz	108	1	22.5	2.6	0	486	.9
-Mr. Salty Dutch	1 oz	110	1	22	3	0	440	na
-Mr. Salty Sticks	1 oz	110	1	22	3	0	660	na
Prickly pear	1 med.	42	.5	9.9	.8	0	6	3.7
Prosciutto								
-Citterio	2 slices	70	4.5	0	8	20	730	0
Prune, dried								
-Sun Sweet	1 1/2 oz	110	0	27	1	0	5	3
Prune juice								
-Mott's All Natural	6 fl oz	136	1	34	1	0	8	na

FOOD	AMOUNT	CAL	FAT	CARB	PROT	CHOL	SOD	FIBER
Pudding, **ready-to-serve** *-Jell-O Pudding Snacks*								
Chocolate	4 oz	160	0	28	3	0	190	0
Chocolate/caramel	4 oz	170	6	28	3	0	190	0
Chocolate/vanilla	4 oz	170	6	28	3	0	190	0
Tapioca	4 oz	170	4	29	3	0	180	0
Vanilla	4 oz	160	5	25	2	0	170	0
-Jell-o Pudding *Free Snacks*								
Chocolate	4 oz	100	0	23	3	0	190	0
Caramel	4 oz	100	0	23	3	0	210	0
Vanilla	4 oz	100	0	23	2	0	240	0
Pudding bar, frozen *-Jell-O Pudding Pops*								
Chocolate	1 bar	80	2	13	2	0	85	na
Chocolate, Double	1 bar	80	2	13	2	0	90	na
Chocolate/Vanilla	1 bar	80	2	13	2	0	70	na
Vanilla	1 bar	80	2	13	2	0	55	na
Puff pastry, frozen *-Pepperidge Farm*	1/6 sheet	170	11	14	3	0	200	1
Pumpkin -fresh, cubed	1/2 c.	15	.1	3.8	.6	0	1	1
Pumpkin butter	1 tsp	12	0	3	0	0	14	na
Pumpkin seeds -roasted	1/3 c.	100	8	3	4	0	5020	2
Q								
Quail, w/skin	1 oz	54	13.1	0	21.4	na	58	0
Quince	1 med.	53	.1	14.1	.4	0	4	1.7
Quinoa *-Arrowhead Mills*	1/4 c.	140	2	25	5	0	0	4

FOOD	AMOUNT	CAL	FAT	CARB	PROT	CHOL	SOD	FIBER
R								
Rabbit								
-domesticated	4 oz	223	9.1	0	33	93	53	0
-wild	4 oz	196	4	0	37.4	139	51	0
Radicchio								
-shredded	1/2 c.	5	.1	.9	.3	0	4	na
Radish								
-sliced	1/2 c.	10	.5	2.1	.6	0	10	.9
Radish, black	1 oz	5	.1	1.8	.3	0	9	.7
Radish, Oriental								
-sliced	1/2 c.	8	.1	1.8	.3	0	9	.7
Radish, white-icicle								
-sliced	1/2 c.	7	.1	1.3	.6	0	8	.4
Raisin								
-Sunmaid								
golden	1/4 c.	130	0	31	1	0	10	2
seedless	1/4 c.	130	0	31	1	0	10	2
Raspberry, fresh								
-black	1/2 c.	49	.9	10.5	1	0	tr	4.4
-red	1/2 c.	35	.3	8.3	.7	0	tr	4.2
Raspberry, frozen								
-Big Valley	2/3 c.	60	0	12	1	0	0	2
Red beans								
-canned								
-Goya	1/2 c.	90	1	19	7	0	350	8
-dried								
-Goya	1/4 c.	70	0	22	9	0	20	14
Refried beans								
-Old El Paso	4 oz	80	2	15	6	5	430	5
-Vegetarian	4 oz	70	1	15	6	0	280	5
Relish								
-Heinz								
Hamburger	1 oz	30	0	7	0	0	325	na
Hot dog	1 oz	35	0	8	0	0	200	na

FOOD	AMOUNT	CAL	FAT	CARB	PROT	CHOL	SOD	FIBER
India	1 oz	35	0	9	0	0	215	na
Piccalilli	1 oz	30	0	7	0	0	145	na
Sweet	1 oz	35	0	9	0	0	205	ma
Rhubarb, fresh								
-diced	1/2 c.	10	.1	2.2	.3	0	1	1.1
Rice, cooked								
-glutinous or sweet	1/2 c.	117	.3	25.4	2.5	0	7	1.2
-white, long grain	1/2 c.	103	.3	22.3	2.2	0	tr	.1
-white, long grain instant	1/2 c.	110	0	23	2	0	0	na
Rice, dry								
-Arrowhead Mills								
basmati, brown	1/4 c.	150	1	33	3	0	0	2
basmati, white	1/4 c.	150	1	34	4	0	0	1
brown, long grain	1/4 c.	150	1	33	3	0	0	2
brown, med. or short grain	1/4 c.	170	1	36	4	0	0	2
-Carolina								
white, enriched	1/4 c.	150	0	35	35	3	0	0
-Fantastic Foods								
arborio	1/4 c.	210	0	45	4	0	0	1
-Uncle Ben's								
white, instant	1/2 c.	190	5	43	3	0	15	1
Rice cakes								
-Quaker								
Apple Cinnamon	1 piece	50	0	11	1	0	0	na
Chocolate Crunch	1 piece	60	1	12	1	0	35	na
Cinnamon Crunch	1 piece	50	0	11	1	0	25	na
Salted	1 piece	35	0	7	1	0	15	na
Unsalted	1 piece	35	0	7	1	0	0	na
Rice drink								
-Rice Dream								
Chocolate	8 fl oz	170	3	36	1	0	115	0
Organic original	8 fl oz	120	2	25	1	0	90	0
Vanilla Lite	8 fl oz	130	2	28	1	0	90	0
Rice flour								
-Arrowhead Mills								
brown	1/4 c.	120	1	27	3	0	0	2
white	1/4 c.	130	.5	28	2	0	0	1

FOOD	AMOUNT	CAL	FAT	CARB	PROT	CHOL	SOD	FIBER
Rockfish	4 oz	107	1.8	0	21.3	39	68	0
Roll								
-Arnold								
dinner	1 piece	50	1	9	2	5	80	1
hamburger	1 piece	120	2	20	4	0	190	2
hot dog	1 piece	110	2	21	4	0	160	1
kaiser	1 piece	170	2	34	5	0	na	na
onion	1 piece	140	3	28	5	0	200	2
potato	1 piece	140	2	25	4	0	210	2
sandwich	1 piece	110	3	18	4	0	170	2
Roll, frozen								
-Pillsbury								
Butterflake	1 piece	140	5	20	3	5	530	na
Crescent	1 piece	100	6	11	2	0	230	na
Roseapple	1 oz	7	.1	1.6	.2	0	tr	.3
Rosemary, dried	1 tsp	4	.2	.8	.1	0	1	.2
Roughy, orange	4 oz	143	8	0	16.7	23	72	0
Rutabaga								
-fresh, cubed	1/2 c.	30	.1	6.9	.7	0	3.5	1.8
Rye flour								
-Arrowhead Mills	1/4 c.	100	1	20	5	0	0	4
S								
Sablefish	4 oz	222	17.4	0	15.2	56	64	0
Safflower seed	1 oz	147	10.9	9.7	4.6	0	0	2.2
Saffron	1 tsp	2	.1	.5	.1	0	1	.1
Sage, ground	1 tsp	2	.1	.4	.1	0	tr	.1
Salad dressing								
-Kraft								
Bacon and Tomato	1 tbsp	70	7	1	0	0	130	na
Blue Cheese	1 tbsp	65	2.5	1	.5	2.5	155	na
Buttermilk	1 tbsp	80	8	1	0	5	120	na

FOOD	AMOUNT	CAL	FAT	CARB	PROT	CHOL	SOD	FIBER
Caesar	1 tbsp	70	7	1	0	0	180	na
Coleslaw	1 tbsp	70	6	4	0	10	200	na
Cucumber	1 tbsp	70	0	4	0	0	270	na
French	1 tbsp	60	6	2	0	0	125	na
Garlic	1 tbsp	50	5	1	0	0	170	na
Italian	1 tbsp	60	6	1	0	0	115	na
Oil and Vinegar	1 tbsp	70	8	1	0	0	210	na
Ranch	1 tbsp	85	9	1	0	2.5	135	na
Russian	1 tbsp	60	5	2	0	5	150	na
Thousand Island	1 tbsp	60	5	2	0	5	150	na
-Kraft Free								
Blue Cheese	2 tbsp	50	0	12	1	0	340	1
French	2 tbsp	50	0	12	0	0	300	1
Honey Dijon	2 tbsp	45	0	10	1	0	340	1
Italian	2 tbsp	10	0	2	0	0	290	0
Ranch	2 tbsp	50	0	11	1	0	310	1
Red Wine Vinegar	2 tbsp	15	0	3	0	0	400	0
Thousand Island	2 tbsp	45	0	11	0	0	300	1
Salmon								
-Atlantic, farmed	4 oz	207	12.3	0	22.6	67	66	0
-Atlantic, wild	4 oz	161	7.2	0	22.5	62	50	0
-Chinook	4 oz	204	11.9	0	22.8	75	53	0
-coho, farmed	4 oz	182	8.7	0	24.1	58	53	0
-coho, wild	4 oz	165	6.7	0	25	51	53	0
-pink	4 oz	132	3.9	0	22.6	59	76	0
-sockeye	4 oz	191	9.7	0	24.2	70	53	0
Salmon, canned								
-Bumble Bee Pink	1/4 c.	90	5	0	12	40	270	0
Salsa								
-Old El Paso Thick								
'n Chunky								
Garden Pepper	2 tbsp	10	0	2	0	0	220	0
Hot	2 tbsp	10	0	2	0	0	230	0
Med.	2 tbsp	10	0	2	0	0	230	0
Mild	2 tbsp	10	0	2	0	0	230	0
Salt								
-kosher	1 tbsp	0	0	0	0	0	6589	0
-noniodized	1 tbsp	0	0	0	0	0	2300	0
-sea	1 tbsp	0	0	0	0	0	2255	0

FOOD	AMOUNT	CAL	FAT	CARB	PROT	CHOL	SOD	FIBER
"Salt," substitute								
-Lawry	1 tbsp	10	.2	1.8	.3	0	2	.4
-Morton	1 tbsp	1	0	.1	0	0	1	na
Salt pork	1 oz	212	22.8	0	1.4	25	404	0
Sandwich sauce								
-Hunt's Manwich	1/4 c.	30	0	6	1	0	360	0
Sardine, canned								
-Haddon House								
in olive oil	1/4 c.	132	9	0	12	48	58	0
spiced	1/4 c.	124	8	0	14	12	110	0
Sauerkraut	1/2 c.	21	.3	4.7	1.2	0	na	3
Sausage								
-Jones Dairy Farm								
Brown and Serve	2 link	180	17	1	6	35	360	0
Italian	1 link	140	11.5	tr	8	44	420	0
pork								
Dinner Link	1 link	150	14	1	6	35	310	0
Little Link	3 link	190	17	1	8	45	420	0
"Sausage,"								
vegetarian, frozen								
-Morningstar Farms								
breakfast links	2 links	60	2.5	2	8	0	340	2
Savory, ground	1 tsp	4	.1	1	.1	0	tr	.2
Scallion								
-fresh, chopped	1/2 c.	18	.1	4.1	.8	0	2	na
Scallop								
-bay or sea, steamed	4 oz	127	1.6	0	26.3	na	na	0
"Scallop," vegetarian								
-Worthington Vegetable								
Skallops	1/2 c.	90	2	4	15	0	430	na
Scallop squash								
-fresh, sliced	1/2 c.	12	.1	2.5	.8	0	1	1.2

FOOD	AMOUNT	CAL	FAT	CARB	PROT	CHOL	SOD	FIBER
Scrapple *-Jones Dairy Farm*	1.5 oz	90	6	5	4	24	230	na
Scrod	4 oz	93	.8	0	20.2	49	62	0
Sea bass	4 oz	110	2.3	0	26.8	47	77	0
Sea trout	4 oz	118	4.1	0	19	94	66	0
Seaweed -agar	1 oz	7	tr	1.9	.2	0	3	.1
-kelp	1 oz	12	.2	2.7	.5	0	66	.4
-laver	1 oz	10	.1	1.4	1.6	0	14	.1
-spirulina	1 oz	8	.1	.7	1.7	0	28	.1
-wakame	1 oz	13	.2	2.6	.9	0	247	.1
Seitan *-Up Country* Chicken Style	1 piece	130	0	12	20	0	470	10
Orginal	4 oz	70	1	0	15	0	60	0
Semolina *-Arrowhead Mills*	1/2 c.	240	1	50	9	0	0	4
Sesame flour -high fat	1 oz	149	10.5	7.6	8.7	0	11	1.8
-partially defatted	1 oz	109	3.4	10	11.5	0	12	1.7
-lowfat	1 oz	95	.5	10.1	14.2	0	11	1.4
Sesame seeds, dry	1/4 c.	210	20	5	7	0	0	5
Shad	4 oz	223	15.6	0	19.2	na	58	0
Shallot -chopped	1 tbsp	7	.1	1.7	.3	0	1	.2
Shark	4 oz	148	5.1	0	23.8	58	90	0
Sherbet *-Sealtest* (all flavors)	1/2 c.	130	1	28	1	5	30	na
Shortening *-Crisco*	1 tbsp	110	12	0	0	0	0	0
Shrimp	4 oz	120	2	1	23	173	168	0

FOOD	AMOUNT	CAL	FAT	CARB	PROT	CHOL	SOD	FIBER
Shrimp, canned	1 c.	148	1.4	.9	31	222	na	0
"Shrimp," imitation	4 oz	115	1.7	10.4	12.1	41	800	0
Smelt, rainbow	4 oz	110	2.8	0	20	80	68	0
Snapper	4 oz	113	1.5	0	23.3	42	73	0
Soda								
-Canada Dry								
Diet Gingerale	8 fl oz	0	0	0	0	0	60	0
Diet Tonic	8 fl oz	0	0	0	0	0	35	0
Gingerale	8 fl oz	100	0	25	0	0	20	0
Seltzer	8 fl oz	0	0	0	0	0	10	0
Seltzer, all flavors	8 fl oz	0	0	0	0	0	10	0
Tonic	8 fl oz	100	0	24	0	0	15	0
-Coca-Cola								
Cherry	8 fl oz	104	0	28	0	0	4	0
Classic	8 fl oz	97	0	27	0	0	9	0
Diet Cherry	8 fl oz	1	0	tr	0	0	4	0
Diet Coke	8 fl oz	1	0	tr	0	0	4	0
-Dr. Pepper								
Diet	8 fl oz	tr	0	tr	0	0	na	0
Regular	8 fl oz	160	0	40	0	0	55	0
-Mountain Dew								
Diet	8 fl oz	2	0	tr	0	0	0	0
Regular	8 fl oz	170	0	46	0	0	70	0
-Mug								
Cream	8 fl oz	122	0	32	0	0	21	0
Diet Cream	8 fl oz	2	0	0	0	0	29	0
Diet Root Beer	8 fl oz	1	0	tr	0	0	26	0
Root Beer	8 fl oz	141	0	29	0	0	26	0
-Pepsi								
Diet	8 fl oz	1	0	tr	0	0	tr	0
Regular	8 fl oz	150	0	41	0	0	35	0
Sole	4 oz	104	1.4	0	21.4	54	92	0
Sorghum, whole -grain	1 c.	650	6.3	143.3	21.7	0	na	4.6
Sorghum syrup	1 tbsp	53	0	14	0	0	na	0
Sorrel, boiled	4 oz	23	.7	3.3	2.1	0	3	.8

FOOD	AMOUNT	CAL	FAT	CARB	PROT	CHOL	SOD	FIBER
Soup, condensed								
-Campbell's								
Asparagus, Cream	1/2 c.	110	7	9	11	5	910	1
Bean w/Bacon	1/2 c.	180	5	25	8	5	890	7
Beef Broth	1/2 c.	15	0	1	0	5	900	0
Broccoli, Cream	1/2 c.	100	6	9	9	5	770	1
Celery, Cream	1/2 c.	110	7	9	11	5	900	1
Cheddar Cheese	1/2 c.	130	8	11	12	20	1080	1
Chicken Broth	1/2 c.	30	2	2	3	5	770	0
Chicken, Cream	1/2 c.	130	8	11	12	10	890	1
Chicken Noodle	1/2 c.	60	2	8	3	15	980	1
Chicken Vegetable	1/2 c.	80	2	12	3	10	940	2
Clam Chowder								
Manhattan	1/2 c.	60	.5	12	1	5	910	2
New England	1/2 c.	100	2.5	15	4	5	980	1
Minestrone	1/2 c.	100	2	16	3	0	960	4
Mushroom, Cream	1/2 c.	110	7	9	11	5	870	1
Onion, Creamy	1/2 c.	110	6	13	9	20	910	1
Potato, Cream	1/2 c.	100	3	14	5	10	890	1
Tomato	1/2 c.	100	2	18	3	0	730	2
Turkey Noodle	1/2 c.	80	2.5	10	4	15	970	1
Turkey Vegetable	1/2 c.	80	2.5	11	4	10	840	2
Vegetable	1/2 c.	80	1.5	14	2	5	920	2
Vegetable, Vegetarian	1/2 c.	70	1	14	2	0	770	2
Soup, mix								
-Campbell's								
Black Bean	1 pkg	250	1.5	48	2	5	1080	6
Chicken	1 pkg	130	2	22	3	25	1290	1
Chicken Noodle	3 tbsp	100	1.5	18	2	10	790	1
Gumbo	1 pkg	170	2	34	3	5	950	2
Lentil, Hearty	1 pkg	240	2.5	42	2	5	1320	7
Noodle, Beef	1 pkg	120	1.5	22	2	20	1260	1
Noodle, Vegetable	1 pkg	150	2	28	3	20	1050	1
Tomato Vegetable	1 pkg	130	2	25	3	15	900	2
-Cup-a-Soup								
Broccoli-Cheese	1 pkg	70	3	8	2	5	550	1
Chicken, Cream of	1 pkg	70	2	12	1	0	640	1
Chicken Noodle	1 pkg	50	1	8	2	10	550	0
Mushroon, Cream	1 pkg	60	2	10	1	0	610	0
Pea	1 pkg	110	3.5	17	3	0	620	3
Tomato	1 pkg	90	1	20	2	0	510	1
Vegetable Chicken	1 pkg	50	1	10	1	10	520	0
-Nissin Ramen								
Noodle, Beef	1 pkg	200	8	27	4	0	1020	1

FOOD	AMOUNT	CAL	FAT	CARB	PROT	CHOL	SOD	FIBER
Noodle, Oriental	1 pkg	200	8	27	4	0	900	1
Noodle, Oriental								
Low fat	1 pkg	150	1	31	3	0	1220	1
Noodle, Chicken	1 pkg	200	8	27	4	0	930	1
Noodle, Pork	1 pkg	200	8	27	4	0	820	1
Noodle, Shrimp	1 pkg	200	8	27	4	0	1070	1
Soup, ready-to-serve								
-Campbell's Chunky								
Bean and Ham	1 c.	190	2	29	3	15	880	0
Beef and Pasta	1 c.	150	3	18	5	20	970	0
Beef Vegetable	1 c.	160	4	18	6	25	900	3
Broccoli Cheese	1 c.	200	12	14	18	25	1120	1
Chicken	1 c.	130	3	12	5	20	950	3
Chicken Noodle	1 c.	130	3	16	5	20	1050	2
Chicken Rice	1 c.	140	3	18	5	25	840	2
Chicken Vegetable	1 c.	90	1	13	2	10	870	3
Clam Chowder								
Manhattan	1 c.	130	4	12	6	5	900	3
New England	1 c.	240	15	21	23	10	980	2
Corn Chowder	1 c.	250	15	18	23	25	870	3
Minestrone	1 c.	140	5	22	8	5	800	2
Pea, Split, w/Ham	1 c.	190	3	27	5	20	1120	3
Vegetable	1 c.	130	3	22	5	0	870	4
Vegetable Beef	1 c.	150	5	17	8	15	870	3
Sour cream								
-Breakstone's	2 tbsp	60	5	1	1	25	15	0
-Breakstone's Half								
and Half	2 tbsp	45	3.5	2	1	15	20	0
-Breakstone's Free	2 tbsp	35	0	6	2	5	25	0
-Friendship	2 tbsp	55	5	1	1	42	15	0
-Friendship Light	2 tbsp	35	2	2	1	8	25	0
Sour cream, nondairy								
-Sour Supreme	2 tbsp	50	5	1	1	0	120	0
Soy drink								
-EdenSoy								
Carob	8 fl oz	150	4	23	6	0	105	0
Original	8 fl oz	130	4	13	10	0	105	0
Vanilla	8 fl oz	150	3	23	6	0	90	0
-Health Valley								
Soy Moo	1 c.	110	0	21	7	0	90	1

FOOD	AMOUNT	CAL	FAT	CARB	PROT	CHOL	SOD	FIBER
Soy flour -*Arrowhead Mills*	1/2 c.	200	9	16	16	0	0	8
Soy protein -concentrate	1 oz	94	.1	8.8	16.5	0	1	1.1
Soy sauce -*Eden*								
tamari	1/2 tsp	2	0	0	0	0	160	0
shoyu	1/2 tsp	2	0	0	0	0	140	0
-*La Choy*	1/2 tsp	2	0	1	1	1	230	1
Soybean	1/4 c.	170	8	14	15	0	0	10
Soybean butter -*Natural Touch*	2 tbsp	170	11	10	6	0	170	1
Soybean flakes	2 oz	250	11	18	20	0	2	8.1
Spaghetti squash -baked	1/2 c.	23	.2	5	.5	0	14	1.1
Spelt flour -*Arrowhead Mills*	1/4 c.	100	.5	24	4	0	0	5
Spinach -fresh, chopped	1/2 c.	7	.1	1.2	.9	0	19	.8
Spinach, canned -*Del Monte*	1/2 c.	30	0	4	2	0	360	2
Spinach, frozen -*Green Giant*	1/2 c.	25	0	3	3	0	240	2
-*Green Giant in* *butter sauce*	1/2 c.	40	1.5	5	2	5	280	2
Spiny lobster	4 oz	127	1.7	2.8	23.4	80	20	0
Split peas, dry -*Arrowhead Mills*	1/4 c.	170	.5	31	12	0	20	7
Sprouts, bean	1 oz	10	.1	1.9	1.1	0	1	na
Squab, w/skin	4 oz	333	27	0	20.9	na	na	0

FOOD	AMOUNT	CAL	FAT	CARB	PROT	CHOL	SOD	FIBER
Squash, summer								
-yellow	1/2 c.	13	.15	2.8	.8	0	.5	.7
-zucchini	1/2 c.	11	.05	2.3	.8	0	.5	.9
Squash, winter								
-acorn squash								
baked, cubed	1/2 c.	57	.1	14.9	1.1	0	4	2.9
-butternut squash								
baked, cubed	1/2 c.	41	.9	10.7	.9	0	4	2.9
-spaghetti squash								
baked	1/2 c.	23	.2	5	.5	0	14	1.1
Squid	4 oz	104	1.6	3.5	17.7	265	50	0
Starfruit	1 med.	42	.4	9.9	.7	0	2	3.4
Steak sauce								
-A1	1 tbsp	12	0	3	0	0	280	na
-French's	1 tbsp	25	0	6	0	0	150	na
-Heinz 57	1 tbsp	16	0	4	0	0	190	0
-Heinz Traditional	1 tbsp	12	0	3	0	0	190	na
-Lee & Perrins	1 tbsp	25	0	6	0	0	135	0
-Maul's	1 tbsp	20	0	5	0	0	250	0
Strawberry	1 c.	55	.7	12.5	1	0	1	3.4
Strawberry, frozen								
-Big Valley	2/3 c.	50	0	12	0	0	0	2
Strawberry milk drink								
(also see "Diet Drinks"								
and "Health Drinks")								
-Nestle Quik mix	1 c.	230	8	32	8	na	140	0
-Nestle Quik	3/4 oz	100	0	24	0	0	0	na
Stuffing								
-Pepperidge Farm								
Apple and Raisin	1 oz	110	1	21	3	na	410	na
Chicken	1 oz	110	1	20	4	na	410	na
Cornbread	1 oz	110	1	22	3	na	320	na
Country Style	1 oz	100	1	21	4	na	400	na
Cube	1 oz	110	1	22	3	na	400	na
Herb, Country								
Garden	1 oz	120	4	18	4	na	300	na
Herb, Seasoned	1 oz	110	1	22	3	na	380	na

FOOD	AMOUNT	CAL	FAT	CARB	PROT	CHOL	SOD	FIBER
Sage and Onion	1 oz	100	1	21	4	0	520	na
Wild Rice and Mushroom	1 oz	130	5	17	4	na	310	na
Stuffing, mix								
-Stove Top								
Beef	1/2 c.	180	9	21	4	0	590	na
Chicken	1/2 c.	180	9	20	4	0	500	na
Chicken w/Rice	1/2 c.	180	9	22	4	0	580	na
Cornbread	1/2 c.	180	9	21	4	0	590	na
Herb	1/2 c.	180	9	20	4	0	580	na
Long Grain and Wild Rice	1/2 c.	180	9	22	4	0	550	na
Mushroom and Onion	1/2 c.	180	9	20	4	0	580	na
Pork	1/2 c.	180	9	20	4	0	560	na
Turkey	1/2 c.	180	9	20	4	0	560	na
Sturgeon								
-fresh	4 oz	180	6.4	0	28.8	na	31	0
-smoked	4 oz	168	2	0	35.2	na	na	0
Sucker	4 oz	105	2.6	0	19	47	45	0
Sugar, beet or cane								
-brown, packed	1 oz	102.6	0	26.5	0	0	8.25	0
-granulated	1 oz	96	0	24.8	0	0	.2	0
-powdered or confectioner's	1/4 c.	120	0	30	0	0	0	0
Sugar, maple	1 oz	99	0	25.5	0	0	4	0
"Sugar," substitute								
-Equal	1 pkt	4	0	1	0	0	0	0
-Sprinkle Sweet	1 tsp	2	0	tr	0	0	1	0
-SugarTwin	1 pkt	3	0	1	0	0	5	0
-Sweet One	1 pkt	4	0	1	0	0	0	0
-Sweet'N Low	1 pkt	4	0	1	0	0	0	0
-Weight Watchers Sweetner	1 pkt	4	0	1	0	0	20	0
Sugar apple	1 c.	234	.8	59.3	4.5	0	28	na

FOOD	AMOUNT	CAL	FAT	CARB	PROT	CHOL	SOD	FIBER
Summer sausage								
-Hillshire Farms								
beef	2 oz	190	17	1	9	na	na	0
beef w/ cheese	2 oz	200	18	1	9	na	na	0
Summer or								
Yellow squash								
-fresh, sliced	1/2 c.	13	.15	2.8	.8	0	.5	.7
Sunflower seed								
-Planters								
dry-roasted	1/4 c.	190	17	6	7	0	230	4
Sunflower seed								
butter	1 tbsp	93	7.6	4.4	3.2	0	1	.8
Sweet potato	1 med.	148	.5	34.1	2.2	0	13	3.9
Sweet and sour sauce								
-Bennett's	1 tbsp	30	0	7	0	0	70	na
-La Choy	1 tbsp	25	1	7	1	0	40	1
-La Choy Duck								
Sauce	1 tbsp	25	1	7	1	0	40	1
-Sauceworks	1 tbsp	25	0	5	0	0	50	na
Swiss chard								
-fresh, chopped	1/2 c.	3	.1	.7	.3	0	38	.3
Swordfish	4 oz	137	4.6	0	22.5	45	102	0
Szechwan sauce								
-La Choy	1 oz	48	.2	12	.1	0	141	0
T								
Tabbouleh mix	1 oz	90	.5	3	19	0	340	5
Taco seasoning mix								
-French's	1/12 pkg	8	0	2	0	0	180	na
-Old El Paso	1/12 pkg	8	1	2	1	0	240	na
Taco shell								
-Chi-Chi's	1 piece	140	7	17	2	0	5	na
-Gebhardt	1 piece	50	2	7	1	0	1	1

FOOD	AMOUNT	CAL	FAT	CARB	PROT	CHOL	SOD	FIBER
-Lawry's	1 piece	50	3	8	.8	0	123	.2
-Old El Paso	1 piece	50	3	6	0	0	95	1.5
-Ortega	1 piece	50	2	8	0	0	5	na
-Rosarita	1 piece	50	2	7	1	0	1	1
-Tio Sancho	1 piece	64	3.1	8.1	1.1	0	1	.5
Tahini								
-Arrowhead Mills	2 tbsp	170	19	5	6	0	5	3
-Joyva	2 tbsp	200	18	3	5	0	75	1
Tamale, canned								
-Derby	2 pieces	160	7	15	8	24	570	1
-Gebhardt	2 pieces	290	22	19	5	54	730	2
-Old El Paso	2 pieces	190	12	16	5	20	380	na
Tamarind	1 med.	5	.1	1.3	.1	0	1	.1
Tangerine	1 med.	39	.2	10	.7	0	2	1.9
Tapioca, pearl, dry	1 tbsp	30	tr	7.3	.1	0	tr	.9
Taramosalata								
-Krinos	1 tbsp	90	10	0	1	15	115	0
Taro								
-fresh, sliced	1/2 c.	56	.1	13.8	.8	0	6	2.1
Taro, Tahitian								
-fresh, sliced	1/2 c.	25	.6	4.3	1.7	0	31	1.1
Tarragon, ground	1 tsp	5	.1	.8	.4	0	1	.1
Tartar sauce								
-Bennett's	1 tbsp	70	7	1	0	5	100	na
-Golden Dipt	1 tbsp	70	7	2	0	10	100	na
-Heinz	1 tbsp	70	7	2	0	3	240	na
-Hellman's	1 tbsp	70	8	0	0	5	220	na
-Sauceworks	1 tbsp	50	5	2	0	5	85	na
Tea, herbal								
-Celestial Seasonings								
Almond Sunset	8 fl oz	3	tr	1	0	0	2	0
Bengal Spice	8 fl oz	5	tr	tr	0	0	3	0
Caffeine Free	8 fl oz	2	tr	1	0	0	5	0
Chamomile	8 fl oz	2	tr	1	0	0	1	0
Cinnamon Apple Spice	8 fl oz	3	tr	tr	0	0	1	0

FOOD	AMOUNT	CAL	FAT	CARB	PROT	CHOL	SOD	FIBER
Cinnamon Rose	8 fl oz	4	tr	1	0	0	1	0
Country Peach Spice	8 fl oz	3	tr	1	0	0	1	0
Cranberry Cove	8 fl oz	2	tr	1	0	0	1	0
Emperor's Choice	8 fl oz	4	tr	1	0	0	2	0
Ginseng Plus	8 fl oz	3	tr	1	0	0	4	0
Grandma's Tummy Mint	8 fl oz	2	tr	tr	0	0	7	0
Lemon Mist	8 fl oz	3	tr	tr	0	0	3	0
Lemon Zinger	8 fl oz	4	tr	1	0	0	1	0
Mama Bear's Cold Care	8 fl oz	6	tr	2	0	0	2	0
Mandarin Orange Spice	8 fl oz	5	tr	1	0	0	2	0
Mellow Mint	8 fl oz	2	tr	tr	0	0	5	0
Mint Magic	8 fl oz	1	tr	tr	0	0	13	0
Orange Zinger	8 fl oz	6	tr	1	0	0	1	0
Peppermint	8 fl oz	2	tr	1	0	0	9	0
Raspberry Patch	8 fl oz	4	tr	1	0	0	1	0
Red Zinger	8 fl oz	4	tr	1	0	0	2	0
Roastaroma	8 fl oz	10	tr	2	0	0	3	0
Sleepytime	8 fl oz	4	tr	1	0	0	2	0
Spearmint	8 fl oz	5	tr	tr	0	0	6	0
Strawberry Fields	8 fl oz	4	tr	1	0	0	1	0
Sunburst C	8 fl oz	3	tr	1	0	0	6	0
Tropical Escape	8 fl oz	1	tr	tr	0	0	7	0
Wild Forest Blackberry	8 fl oz	2	tr	1	0	0	1	0
Tea, iced								
-canned								
Lipton Brisk	8 fl oz	160	0	39	0	0	10	0
Shasta	8 fl oz	136	0	34	0	0	58	0
-mix								
Lipton, w/sugar	8 fl oz	60	0	14	0	0	0	0
Nestea Ice Teasers	8 fl oz	6	0	1	0	0	0	0
Nestea Presweet	8 fl oz	70	0	19	0	0	0	0
Tempeh								
-Light Life								
3 Grain	4 oz	190	4	25	12	0	17	6
Soy	4 oz	182	6	9	24	0	12	1
Wild Rice	4 oz	190	4	25	12	0	20	7
Tempura batter mix								
-Golden Dipt	1/4 c.	120	0	15	2	na	160	na

FOOD	AMOUNT	CAL	FAT	CARB	PROT	CHOL	SOD	FIBER
Teriyaki marinade								
-Lawry's	2 tbsp	72	.4	11	6.4	0	7100	.2
Teriyake sauce								
-La Choy	1/2 tsp	5	1	1	1	0	290	1
-La Choy Lite	1/2 tsp	5	1	1	1	0	85	1
Thyme, ground	1 tsp	4	.1	.9	.1	0	1	.3
Tilefish	4 oz	108	2.6	0	19.9	na	60	0
Toaster muffins and pastries								
-Kellogg's Pop-Tarts								
Apple Cinnamon	1 piece	210	6	37	2	0	170	1
Blueberry	1 piece	210	6	37	2	0	210	0
Blueberry, Frosted	1 piece	200	6	37	2	0	210	0
Brown Sugar-Cinnamon	1 piece	210	8	33	3	0	200	0
Cherry	1 piece	210	6	37	2	0	220	0
Chocolate Fudge	1 piece	200	5	37	3	0	220	0
Chocolate Graham	1 piece	210	6	37	3	0	210	0
Raspberry	1 piece	200	5	37	2	0	210	0
Strawberry	1 piece	210	6	37	2	0	210	0
-Pillsbury Toaster Strudel								
Apple	1 piece	200	9	26	3	5	190	na
Cinnamon	1 piece	200	10	23	5	5	200	na
Strawberry	1 piece	190	9	26	3	5	200	na
-Thomas' Toast-r-Cakes								
Banana Nut	1 piece	110	4	17	2	10	200	1
Blueberry	1 piece	100	3	17	2	10	170	1
Chocolate Chip	1 piece	100	4	15	2	10	150	1
Corn	1 piece	120	4	20	2	10	190	1
Raisin Bran	1 piece	100	3	18	2	10	180	1
Tofu								
-Nasoya								
extra firm	3 oz	90	5	1	9.1	0	10	0
firm	3 oz	80	4	2	8	0	10	0
silken	3 oz	50	2	2	4.5	0	10	0
soft	3 oz	60	3	2	6.6	0	10	0

FOOD	AMOUNT	CAL	FAT	CARB	PROT	CHOL	SOD	FIBER
Tofu patty, frozen								
-Natural Touch								
Garden	1 patty	120	4	8	11	0	300	na
-Natural Touch								
Okara	1 patty	160	10	7	11	0	420	na
Tomatillo	1 med.	11	.4	2	.3	0	tr	.6
Tomato								
-red, fresh	1 med.	27	.2	5.8	1.4	0	4	1
Tomato, canned								
-Contadina								
Crushed	1/4 c.	20	0	4	1	0	150	1
Italian paste	2 tbsp	40	1	7	1	0	320	1
Italian Pear	1/2 c.	25	0	4	1	0	220	1
Italian Stewed	1/2 c.	40	0	8	1	0	260	1
Mexican Stewed	1/2 c.	40	0	9	1	0	220	1
Paste	2 tbsp	30	0	6	2	0	20	1
Peeled Whole	1/2 c.	25	0	4	1	0	220	1
Puree	1/4 c.	20	0	4	1	0	15	tr
Stewed	1/2 c.	40	0	9	1	0	250	1
-Muir Glen Organic								
Chunky Sauce	1/4 c.	20	0	4	1	0	160	1
Crushed w/Basil	1/4 c.	25	0	4	1	0	85	1
Diced	1/4 c.	25	0	4	1	0	290	1
Paste	2 tbsp	30	0	6	2	0	20	1
Puree	1/4 c.	20	0	5	1	0	20	1
Sauce	1/4 c.	20	0	5	1	0	190	1
Stewed	1/2 c.	30	0	7	1	0	290	tr
Whole, Peeled	1/2 c.	30	0	5	1	0	260	1
Tomato, green	1 med.	30	.3	6.3	1.5	0	16	1.8
Tomato, pickled	1 oz	5	0	1	0	0	320	1
Tomato, sundried								
-Sonoma	3 halves	15	0	3	1	0	5	1
Tomato juice								
-Campbell's	8 fl oz	50	0	9	1	0	860	1
Tortellini								
-Contadina								
3 Cheese	3/4 c.	260	6	41	11	35	290	1

FOOD	AMOUNT	CAL	FAT	CARB	PROT	CHOL	SOD	FIBER
Mushroom	1 c.	290	3	49	11	45	250	2
Spinach	3/4 c.	260	6	39	13	55	390	3
Tortilla								
-*Goya*								
corn	2 pieces	120	1.5	26	2	0	0	3
flour	1 piece	110	0	2.5	18	3	290	3
Trout								
-rainbow, farmed	4 oz	156	6.1	0	23.7	67	40	0
-rainbow, wild	4 oz	135	3.9	0	23.2	67	35	0
Tuna								
-bluefin	4 oz	163	5.6	0	26.5	43	44	0
-skipjack	4 oz	117	1.2	0	25	53	42	0
-yellowfin	4 oz	123	1.1	0	26.5	51	42	0
Tuna, canned, drained								
-*Bumble Bee*								
chunck light, oil	2 oz	110	6	0	13	30	250	0
chunck light, water	2 oz	60	.5	0	13	30	250	0
solid white, oil	2 oz	90	3	0	14	25	250	0
solid white, water	2 oz	70	1	0	15	25	250	0
"Tuna," vegetarian								
-frozen								
Worthington								
Tuno	1/2 c.	80	6	2	6	0	290	1
Turbot, European	4 oz	108	3.4	0	18.2	na	170	0
Turkey								
-breast, raw	4 oz	190	9	0	24	70	60	0
-ground	4 oz	190	12	0	20	90	140	0
-leg, raw	4 oz	160	8	0	22	85	85	0
-roasted w/skin	4 oz	236	11	0	31.9	93	77	0
"Turkey," vegetarian								
-frozen, smoked								
Worthington	3 slices	140	10	3	10	0	620	2
Turkey bacon								
-*Louis Rich*	1/2 oz	30	2.5	0	2	10	190	0

FOOD	AMOUNT	CAL	FAT	CARB	PROT	CHOL	SOD	FIBER
Turkey dishes, frozen								
-Lean Cuisine								
Glazed	1 pkg	250	6	36	14	30	590	5
Homestyle	1 pkg	230	6	26	18	50	590	3
Pot Pie	1 pkg	300	9	34	20	50	590	3
Roasted Breast and								
Stuffing	1 pkg	290	4	48	16	25	530	0
-Weight Watchers								
Breast, Stuffed	1 pkg	230	5	28	17	15	680	6
Turkey, giblets								
-simmered	4 oz	169	11	1.1	14.9	na	na	0
Turkey gravy								
-Franco-American	1/4 c.	25	1	3	2	5	290	0
Turkey nuggets								
-breaded								
Louis Rich	4 pcs	260	16	15	13	35	640	0
Turkey sausage								
-Louis Rich								
links	2 links	90	6	0	11	45	470	0
Italian	4 oz	170	9	1	20	70	800	0
Smoked	2 oz	80	5	2	9	35	500	0
Turmeric, dried	1/4 tsp	2	0	.4	.1	0	1	.1
Turnip								
-fresh, cubed	1/2 c.	19.5	.15	4.3	.6	0	32	1.2
Turnip greens								
-boiled, chopped	1/2 c.	14	.15	2.6	1.6	0	na	.7
Tzatziki	2 tbsp	60	5	1	3	5	115	0
V								
Veal, roasted								
-ground	4 oz	195	8.6	0	27.6	117	94	0
-leg, lean only	4 oz	170	3.8	0	31.8	117	77	0
-loin, lean only	4 oz	198	7.9	0	29.8	120	109	0
-rib, lean only	4 oz	201	8.4	0	29.2	130	110	0
-shoulder, arm								
lean only	4 oz	186	6.6	0	29.6	124	110	0

FOOD	AMOUNT	CAL	FAT	CARB	PROT	CHOL	SOD	FIBER
-shoulder, blade lean only	4 oz	194	7.8	0	29.1	135	116	0
-shoulder, whole lean only	4 oz	193	7.5	0	29.3	129	110	0
-sirloin	4 oz	191	7.1	0	29.8	118	96	0
Vegetable juice								
-V-8	8 fl oz	50	0	10	1	0	620	1
-V-8 Low Sodium	8 fl oz	60	0	11	1	0	140	2
Venison	3 oz	107	3.4	0	17.9	95	na	0
Vienna sausage								
-Hormel	2 oz	150	14	1	6	45	460	0
-Libby's	3 links	150	14	1	6	45	460	0
Vinegar								
-Balsamic	1 tbsp	5	0	2	0	0	0	0
-Hain Cider	1 tbsp	2	0	4	0	0	1	0
-Heinz								
apple cider	1 tbsp	2	0	0	0	0	1	0
malt	1 tbsp	4	0	0	0	0	5	0
white, distilled	1 tbsp	2	0	0	0	0	0	0
wine	1 tbsp	4	0	0	0	0	0	0
-Ka-Me								
Chinese Seasoned	1 tbsp	5	0	1	0	0	60	0
Rice Wine Chinese	1 tbsp	5	0	1	0	0	0	0
Rice Wine Japanese	1 tbsp	0	0	1	0	0	0	0
Seasoned Rice Wine Japanese	1 tbsp	10	0	3	0	0	180	0
W								
Waffles, frozen								
-Downyflake								
Blueberry	1 piece	90	2	16	1	0	285	na
Buttermilk	1 piece	85	2	15	2	0	315	na
Crisp & Healthy	1 piece	80	1	16	2	0	180	1
Hot-N-Buttery	1 piece	90	3	13.5	2	na	310	na
Plain	1 piece	60	1.5	10	3	0	280	na
-Eggo								
Apple Cinnamon	1 piece	130	5	18	3	15	250	0
Blueberry	1 piece	130	5	18	8	12	250	0

FOOD	AMOUNT	CAL	FAT	CARB	PROT	CHOL	SOD	FIBER
Buttermilk	1 piece	120	5	16	3	15	220	0
Homestyle	1 piece	120	5	16	3	15	250	0
Minis	4 pieces	90	3	14	2	10	190	0
Nut and Honey	1 piece	130	6	17	3	15	250	0
Nutri-Grain	2 pieces	180	6	28	6	0	430	0
Walnuts								
-Skinners	1/4 c.	170	17	5	4	0	0	1
Walnut topping								
-Smucker's	2 tbsp	130	1	27	2	0	0	na
Water chestnut								
-Chinese	1 oz	17	tr	4.2	.3	0	4.3	na
-canned								
La Choy Sliced	1/4 c.	18	1	4	1	0	3	1
La Choy Whole	4 med.	14	1	4	1	0	2	1
Watercress								
-fresh, chopped	1/2 c.	3.5	.1	.5	.4	0	7	.4
Watermelon								
-fresh, diced	1/2 c.	21	.1	5.1	.4	0	1	.4
Wheat, whole-grain								
-durum	1 c.	650	4.7	136.6	26.3	0	3	na
-hard red	1 c.	631	3.7	130.6	29.6	0	4	24.2
-hard white	1 c.	656	3.3	145.7	21.7	0	na	na
-soft white	1 c.	571	3.3	126.6	18	0	na	na
Wheat bran	1 oz	61	1.2	18.3	4.4	0	1	12.1
Wheat flour								
-Arrowhead Mills								
white	1/3 c.	160	.5	33	5	0	0	0
whole wheat	1/4 c.	130	.5	25	5	0	0	4
-Gold Medal								
white, all-purpose	1 c.	400	1	87	11	0	0	na
white, bread	1 c.	400	1	83	14	0	0	na
white, self-rising	1 c.	380	1	83	9	0	1520	na
whole grain	1 c.	350	2	78	16	0	0	10
-Pillsbury's Best								
white, all-purpose	1 c.	400	1	86	12	0	0	3
white, bread	1 c.	400	2	83	14	0	0	2
white, self-rising	1 c.	380	1	84	9	0	1290	2

FOOD	AMOUNT	CAL	FAT	CARB	PROT	CHOL	SOD	FIBER
whole grain	1 c.	400	2	80	15	0	10	12
-*Wondra*	1 c.	400	1	87	11	0	0	na
Wheat germ	1 tbsp	23	.7	3	1.8	0	tr	1
Wheat gluten	1 oz	100	1	9	15	0	1	.9
Whelk	4 oz	156	.5	8.8	27	74	234	0
Whipped topping								
-*Cool Whip*								
Extra Creamy	2 tbsp	30	2	2	0	0	5	0
Lite	2 tbsp	20	1	2	0	0	0	0
Nondairy	2 tbsp	25	1.5	2	0	0	0	0
White beans								
-*Goya*								
canned	1/2 c.	100	2	20	6	0	360	6
dried	1/4 c.	70	0	22	8	0	15	14
White rice flour								
-*Arrowhead Mills*	1/4 c.	130	.5	28	2	0	0	1
Whitefish	4 oz	153	6.7	0	21.7	68	58	0
Whiting	4 oz	102	1.5	0	20.8	76	82	0
Wild rice								
-dry	1 c.	282.5	.6	60.3	11.3	0	5.5	4
Wine								
-dessert or aperitif	1 fl oz	41	0	2.3	tr	0	1	0
-dry or table	1 fl oz	25	0	1.2	tr	0	1	0
Wine, cooking								
-*Holland House*								
Marsala	1 fl oz	9	0	2.3	0	0	186	0
red	1 fl oz	6	0	1.5	0	0	186	0
sherry	1 fl oz	5	0	1.2	0	0	186	0
vermouth	1 fl oz	2	0	1	0	0	186	0
white	1 fl oz	2	0	1	0	0	186	0
Winged bean								
-raw, sliced	1/2 c.	11	.2	1	1.5	0	1	.6
-dry	1/2 c.	372	14.9	38	27	0	35	14.1

FOOD	AMOUNT	CAL	FAT	CARB	PROT	CHOL	SOD	FIBER
Wolf fish	4 oz	109	2.7	0	19.9	52	97	0
Wonton wrapper								
-Nasoya	5 pieces	90	0	13	9	0	130	0
Worcestershire Sauce								
-French's	1 tbsp	8	1	2	1	0	180	0
-Heinz	1 tbsp	6	0	1	0	0	170	0
-Lea & Perrins	1 tsp	5	0	1	0	0	65	0
-Lea & Perrins White Wine	1 tsp	4	0	1	0	0	25	0

Y

FOOD	AMOUNT	CAL	FAT	CARB	PROT	CHOL	SOD	FIBER
Yam								
-fresh, baked	1/2 c.	79	.1	18.8	1	0	6	2.7
Yard-long bean								
-fresh, sliced	1/2 c.	22	.2	3.8	1.3	0	2	na
Yeast								
-Fleischmann's								
active dry	1 pkg	20	0	3	3	0	10	na
fresh active	1 pkg	15	0	2	2	0	5	na
household	1/2 oz	15	0	2	2	0	5	na
RapidRise	1 pkg	20	0	3	3	0	10	na
Yellowtail	4 oz	166	6	0	26.3	na	44	0
Yogurt								
-Breyers								
Cherry, Black	8 oz	230	2	44	9	20	130	0
Coffee	8 oz	220	3	38	10	20	125	0
Peach	8 oz	230	2	43	9	20	125	0
Pineapple	8 oz	230	2	43	9	20	125	0
Raspberry	8 oz	230	2	43	9	20	125	0
Strawberry	8 oz	220	2	43	9	20	125	0
Vanilla	8 oz	220	3	38	10	20	135	0
-Colombo Nonfat								
Blueberry	8 oz	100	0	16	7	5	110	0
Peach	8 oz	100	0	16	7	5	110	0
Raspberry	8 oz	100	0	16	7	5	110	0
Strawbeery	8 oz	100	0	16	7	5	110	0

FOOD	AMOUNT	CAL	FAT	CARB	PROT	CHOL	SOD	FIBER
Vanilla	8 oz	170	0	34	8	5	130	0
-Dannon Nonfat								
Blueberry	8 oz	100	0	20	9	5	140	0
Lemon	8 oz	100	0	17	9	5	140	0
Peach	8 oz	100	0	18	9	5	140	0
Raspberry	8 oz	100	0	39	8	5	135	0
Strawberry-Banana	8 oz	100	0	18	9	5	140	0
Vanilla	8 oz	100	0	17	9	5	140	0
-Light N' Lively Free 50 Cal								
all fruit flavors	1 c.	50	0	8	5	5	60	0
Yogurt, frozen								
-Ben & Jerry Nonfat								
Cappuccino	1/2 c.	150	0	30	5	0	80	0
Chocolate	1/2 c.	130	0	29	3	0	50	0
Coffee Fudge	1/2 c.	140	0	31	4	0	55	0
Rasberry, Black	1/2 c.	140	0	32	3	0	55	0
Vanilla Fudge	1/2 c.	160	0	35	5	0	85	0
Yogurt bar								
-Frozfruit Nonfat								
all flavors	1 bar	90	0	20	3	0	55	na
Yogurt shake, frozen								
-Weight Watchers								
Chocolate	7.5 fl oz	220	1	44	8	5	140	na
Yuca	4 oz	77	.2	38.6	1.2	0	2	na
Z								
Zucchini								
p-fresh, sliced	1/2 c.	11	.05	2.3	.8	0	.5	.9